WITH EMILIE BARNES OF
MORE HOURS IN MY DAY

Desserts

With Lowfat &
Allergy Alternatives

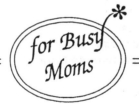

for Busy
Moms

2nd Edition

SUE GREGG

Eating Better Cookbooks

PUBLICATIONS BY SUE GREGG AND EMILIE BARNES

The 15 Minute Meal Planner (Harvest House, 1994)
Meals in Minutes (Harvest House, 1993)

Sue Gregg (Eating Better Cookbooks)
   Main Dishes, 2nd edition
   Soups & Muffins, 2nd edition
   Casseroles, 2nd edition
   Lunches & Snacks, 2nd edition
   Breakfasts, 2nd edition
   Desserts, 2nd edition
   Master Index & Menu Planner
   Eating Better with Sue, Video
   Eating Better with Sue Cooking Course Workbook
   Eating Better with Sue Cooking Course Leader's Guide
   Yeast Breads, 2nd edition
   Holiday Menus
   The Creative Recipe Organizer

Emilie Barnes (Harvest House)
   More Hours in My Day
   Survival for Busy Women
   The Creative Home Organizer
   The 15 Minute Organizer
   The Holiday Organizer
   Growing a Great Marriage
   Things Happen When Women Care
   The Daily Planner
   The Spirit of Loveliness

Published and distributed by
EATING BETTER COOKBOOKS, 8830 Glencoe Drive
Riverside, California 92503-2135   (909) 687-5491

Copyright © 1996 by Rich and Sue Gregg
Second Edition printed December 1994, January 1996
ISBN 1-878272-08-X

DISCLAIMER

This cookbook is designed to provide information relating to the subject matter covered. It is sold with the understanding that the publisher and author are not engaged in rendering medical, nutritional, dietary, or other professional services. If expert assistance is required, the reader should seek the services of a competent medical professional.

This cookbook does not cover or reprint all of the information on the subject available to the author, publisher, or the reader. Research in the field of nutrition often seems conflicting, and when hyped by media and advertising, contradictory and confusing. You are urged to read all the available material, to inform yourself as much as possible about nutrition and food preparation, and then with the advice of competent professionals to tailor the information to your personal needs.

Health is not achieved through one shot schemes, potions, or pills. It is not acquired through diet alone. Anyone who decides to pursue it must expect to invest time, effort, and discipline. We are reminded, however, that even those who inherit or achieve even the best health do not live forever . . . *man is destined to die once...(Heb. 9:27)*. Therefore, the reader is urged not just to prepare for the immediate, but also to discover the Creator's eternal plan (see *The Best Comes Last*, pp. 160-161).

With every edition and printing of this cookbook an effort is made to make the information as accurate, complete, and up-to-date as possible. However, experience tells us that mistakes are inevitable in content, data calculations, and typography. This cookbook should be used only as a general guide and not as the ultimate source of information on food preparation and nutrition.

The purpose of this cookbook is to model and motivate, to educate and entertain. The author and the publisher shall have neither liability nor responsibility to any person or entity with respect to any loss or damage caused, alleged to be caused, directly or indirectly, by the information contained in this book.

If you do not wish to be bound by the above, you may return this book to the publisher for a full refund.

What others are saying...

I go all the way now with "Eating Better." My energy level has increased greatly! Another benefit has been a 20 lb. weight loss!
            Betty Lamb, Jenison, Michigan

Your recipes have really encouraged my cooking. My husband is pleased. Happy husband means a happy wife!
            Christa, San Bernardino, California

You have done an excellent job presenting healthful eating with taste appeal, ease of preparation, familiar dishes, color, and beauty with thanksgiving to our God and Creator.
            Kathleen Hoffman, Somerset, Wisconsin

I love your approach. You use "real people" food but it's done in a healthy way.   Lori Leeke, Plano, Texas

Your cookbooks have changed my life. Our weekly food budget has decreased from $125 to $70. I can't thank you enough.
            Sheila Preston, Ontario, Canada

Your cookbooks are all I ever use. The recipes are hassle-free to make. No special ingredients to buy. They are healthy and taste great! My family loves them. Thank you for writing such wonderful books!
            Chris Gordon, Everett, Washington

We've had lots of allergy problems and have been on rotation diets, vegetarian diets, combination diets, no dairy diets...Cooking became a trial to be put off as long as possible. Your books are sensible...We have only begun, but so far it is all I'd hoped for and more.
            Sherry Schindler, Bartlesville, Oklahoma

I've been using the Eating Better Cookbooks for 1½ years. After 10 years of marriage, what a blessing to hear "This is good! This is really good!" Recipe after recipe! Praise God!
            Kathie Moran, Sacramento, California

I love the cookbooks and menu planner! I've been converting recipes and using various health cookbooks for years, but these are far superior! Thanks!   Sara, Pasadena, Texas

Thank God for bringing you into our lives. When my family asks, "Whose recipe?" and I answer, "Sue Gregg's."
            Johnne Neiner, Pittsfield, Massachusetts

Contents

Cook's Prayer

O LORD, our God, Maker of Heaven and Earth's Land,
You made the wheat, the germ, the bran--
nutrient and fiber-rich for the strength of man,
and all our children;
Cheeses 'n chicken, fish, beef, 'n dairy--
A little goes a long way to refresh the weary.

And vegetables countless--nutrient-packed treasure,
Succulent fruits for dessert--What delightful pleasure!
And nuts 'n seeds for essential fats in good measure.

Beans 'n peas for more protein and fiber, please!
With plenteous water to cook them,
Poured out by the Lord of Seas.
What great gifts, these!
Your store of food in all colors, shapes, and sizes
Are ever full of nutrient and taste surprises!

Honey dripping from the comb,
of this sweet offering could be written a tome.
Spices and herbs to jazz up flavor,
Even salt and egg yolks we count not totally
out of your favor!

Now, O LORD, our God,
Help us to put your bounty together
In balance and wholeness that we might eat better,
For bodies stronger,
And minds sharper;
For spirits assisted,
And service enlisted,
To sow the seed; to reap the harvest
From the nearest land to the farthest.

Planning
for Desserts

In the house of the wise are stores of choice food and oil . . .
Proverbs 21:20

Planning for Desserts

Commercial or Home-Made?

How easy it is these days to buy donuts, pie or ice cream at the market. What's in desserts and packaged mixes? How do you evaluate what's good and what isn't?

The following is a list of different ways nutritional information is printed on package labels. In what order would you rate them as an adequate guide to nutritional value?

a) Product Name

b) Brand

c) Nutritional information written on front of the package

d) Where purchased

e) Nutrition Facts label

f) Ingredients list

Compare the labels of two brands crackers on the chart, p. 6. Which information do you think is the best guide to the nutritional quality? The name of the product in this case obviously communicates no difference. Titles such as *Fat Free Oatmeal Cookies* or *Low Sodium Wheat Thins* imply a nutritional benefit. A name, however, usually highlights only the main selling point. This is also true for highlighted nutritional information on the front of the package. It does not give a complete picture of the product's nutritional quality. The brand name may or may not be helpful. Some companies such as *Health Valley* and *Arrowhead Mills* are committed to high nutritional standards. In most cases health food stores are a better starting place for packaged foods of higher nutritional value, but the nutritional standards are not necessarily consistent (and truly good taste is often lacking).

Now compare the two Nutrition Facts labels (It might be helpful to find a package of another food in your cupboard that includes the Daily Values portion of the label to make this comparison). By observing only the Nutrition Facts label, which product would you rate higher in nutritonal value? What percentage of calories come from fat in a serving of Brand #1? Of Brand #2? If you answered 23% fat for Brand #1 and 12.5% fat for Brand #2 you answered correctly. If you answered 5% fat for Brand #1 and 2% fat for Brand #2 you answered in reference to Daily Values, not in terms of how many calories of a cracker serving come from fat. Are you beginning to get a little confused? For a more comprehensive understanding of the new standardized Nutrition Facts Label see **The 15 Minute Meal Planner**, pp. 292-302. Most people would rate the crackers from the supermarket (Brand #2) as higher in

BRAND #1

Product Name: Honey Grahams
Brand : Mi-Del
Front of Package: 100% Whole Wheat

Where Purchased: Health Food Store

Nutrition Facts

Serving Size 2 crackers (30 g)*
Servings Per Container 16

Amount per Serving

Calories 110	Calories from Fat 25

	% Daily Value**
Total Fat 3g	5%
Saturated Fat 0 g	0%
Cholesterol 0mg	0%
Sodium 190 mg	8%
Total Carbohydrate 22g	7%
Dietary Fiber 2g	8%
Sugars 6 g	
Protein 2g	

Vitamin A 0%	Vitamin C 0%
Calcium 0%	Iron 4%

Ingredients:

Whole wheat flour, honey,
unsulfured molasses, soybean oil,
leavening (sodium bicarbonate,
ammonium bicarbonate), salt,
lecithin, oil of lemon

BRAND #2

Product Name: Honey Graham Selects
Brand : Keebler
Front of Package: Low Fat
    1½ grams of Fat Per Serving
Where Purchased: Supermarket

Nutrition Facts

Serving Size 9 crackers (31 g)*
Servings Per Container 13

Amount per Serving

Calories 120	Calories from Fat 15

	% Daily Value**
Total Fat 1.5g	2%
Saturated Fat 0.5 g	3%
Cholesterol 0mg	0%
Sodium 210 mg	8%
Total Carbohydrate 22g	9%
Dietary Fiber 1g	4%
Sugars 6 g	
Protein 2g	

Vitamin A 0%	Vitamin C 0%
Calcium 0%	Iron 6%

Ingredients:

Enriched flour [wheat flour, niacin,
reduced iron, thiamine mononitrate
(vitamin B1) and riboflavin (vitamin
B2)], sugar, graham flour, honey,
molasses, vegetable shortening
(partially hydrogenated soybean
and/or cottonseed oils), salt,
emulsifiers (mono-& diglycerides,
soy lecithin), sodium bicarbonate,
colored with annatto and tumeric)

*Serving size of these two brands are approximately the same, within 1 gram
in weight. Eight crackers of Keebler Brand equal 2 crackers of Mi-Del Brand.

**The Daily Values portion of the Nutrition Facts chart is not shown here; it is
the same on all food products.

nutritional value than Brand #1 from the health food store. Read the ingredients label of each brand and see if you come to the same conclusion. Consider the quality of fat, flour, and sugars used in each brand plus chemical additions. Which brand do you think has a better balance of nutritional value? I believe the ingredients list gives a clearer and truer picture. Learn to distinguish ingredients of low nutritional quality from those of high nutritional value. If you survey the ingredients used in several ready-made commercial desserts and dessert mixes in the supermarket, you will find the following ingredients used repeatedly (as in Brand #2):

~hydrogenated or partially hydrogenated vegetable fats or oil (often animal fat such as fat from lard, beef)

~corn syrup and/or white sugar, dextrose

~enriched wheat flour (usually bleached)

You will find these ingredients in all types of cakes, cake mixes, cookies, cookie mixes, crackers, frozen pies, frozen desserts, and pudding mixes in the supermarkets. Even fat-free products still contain refined white flour, refined sugars, additives, preservatives, and leavenings that contain aluminum. Sugar-free offerings contain artificial sweeteners such as aspartame or NutraSweet.

Commercial desserts of high nutritional quality in supermarkets are almost nonexistent. The following tips will help you stay committed to making your own:

~ Keep a good stock of basic non-perishable ingredients for desserts on hand (restock items before they run out).

~ Have a few dessert recipes for special occasions that are especially well-liked.

~ If a dessert freezes well, prepare and freeze it well in advance of serving time.

~ Prepare a dessert in stages. For example, chop nuts, measure out ingredients, grease pans the night before or in the morning; complete dessert the next day or later the same day.

~ Consider some of the desserts of higher nutritional quality offered at health food stores to occasionally fill in the gaps.

Why spend money on what is not bread, and your labor on what does not satisfy? Listen, listen to me, and eat what is good. Isaiah 55:2

WHAT ABOUT HEALTH FOOD STORE ALTERNATIVES?

More and more packaged cookies of higher nutritional value can be found in health food stores. These usually contain whole grain flours, fruit concentrates, honey, molasses or some other natural sugar for sweetener, a better quality of oil such as canola oil that is not hydrogenated, natural flavors, etc. They are expensive ranging from about $.11-$.14 per cookie as compared to $.06-$.15 per cookie for recipes in this book. On the other hand, commercial *fat free* cookies are considerably higher in cost, ranging from $.29-$.35 per cookie as compared to $.06-$.12 for fat free recipes in **Desserts**. See guidelines on pp. 32-33.

In most cases you will find healthy prepackaged desserts or dessert mixes more costly than preparing your own and not as tasty. And whether in supermarket or health food store, remember to read the ingredients list.

Alternative Ingredients for Allergies

Ingredients used repeatedly that cause allergy problems for many include wheat flour, eggs, milk, chocolate, and corn (in baking powder and cornstarch). The recipes in **Desserts** offer alternatives:

~ Replace wheat flour with barley flour or a combination of barley flour, rice flour, and oat bran. Kamut, spelt, and nut flours are other alternatives. See pp. 20-22.

~ To replace eggs, see p. 39.

~ In baking, the following liquids are generally interchangeable: milk, buttermilk, yogurt, kefir, nut milk, soy milk, rice milk, fruit juice. Some adjustment may be needed in amount added, and the resulting texture may vary.
Add a tablespoon vinegar to soy or rice milk to replace buttermilk. Soy milk or rice milk can be used in puddings; *Better Than Milk* tofu beverage works best. See p. 39.

~ Replace baking powder with low sodium baking powder.

~ Replace cornstarch with arrowroot powder. See p. 44-45.

~ Replace chocolate or cocoa with carob powder. See p. 41.

"Everything is permissible to me"--but not
everything is beneficial. 1 Corinthians 6:12

Choosing Ingredient Alternatives

I use the chart below as guideline for choosing dessert ingredients for higher nutritional quality or to meet allergy needs. This does not mean that I never use some ingredients in the first column in **Desserts**. For example, I sometimes use battery eggs (eggs from caged non-fertile, non-range fed chickens), and I often use cornstarch and chocolate. On the other hand, I try to avoid all the sugars listed in the first column along with white flour, margarine, and shortening.

IN PLACE OF:	USE:
SUGARS white sugar (cane) brown sugar powdered (confectioner's) sugar raw sugar (e.g. *Yellow D*) corn syrup *Equal* (*NutraSweet*, aspartame)	SUGARS *(p. 23)* honey whole cane sugar (*Sucanat*) fruit concentrates date sugar molasses, unsulfured crystalline fructose *FruitSource*
FLOUR/GRAINS white flour (wheat) graham crackers (refined) refined grain breakfast cereals	FLOUR/GRAINS *(p. 19)* whole wheat pastry flour whole wheat flour brown rice flour barley flour oats, oat flour, oat bran Kamut spelt other whole grains nut flours whole wheat grahams whole grain cereals
FATS margarine shortening lard polyunsaturated oils	FATS *(p. 32)* butter, unsalted canola oil olive oil fat substitute products

IN PLACE OF:	USE:
DAIRY PRODUCTS	DAIRY PRODUCTS *(p. 39)*
whole milk, homogenized	raw certified milk nonfat (skim) or lowfat milk buttermilk soy milk (non-dairy) rice milk (non-dairy)
instant nonfat dry milk	non-instant nonfat dry milk
yogurt with gelatin, without live (active) cultures full fat yogurt, homogenized	yogurt with live cultures nonfat yogurt full fat yogurt, pasteurized lowfat yogurt
whipping cream	raw certified whipping cream
sour cream	nonfat sour cream light sour cream
cream cheese	light cream cheese *Neufchatel* cheese ricotta cheese (skim milk)
EGGS	EGGS *(p. 39)*
eggs, battery (from caged chickens)	eggs, fertile or range-fed egg substitutes
LEAVENINGS, THICKENERS	LEAVENINGS, THICKENERS *(p. 44)*
baking powder	low sodium baking powder *Rumford* baking powder baking soda
cornstarch	arrowroot powder
jello	unflavored gelatine

Good understanding wins favor. . . Proverbs 13:15

IN PLACE OF:	USE:
FRUITS/JUICES	FRUITS/JUICES (p. 39)
sweetened juices	unsweetened juices
sweetened canned fruits	canned fruits in own juices
	or fresh fruits
sweetened frozen fruits	unsweetened frozen fruits
dried fruits, sulfured	dried fruits, unsulfured
date dices, sugar coated	date dices, oat flour coated
sugar sweetened jams	100% or all-fruit spreads
	or honey sweetened spreads
NUTS & SEEDS	NUTS & SEEDS (p. 43)
roasted	unroasted or home roasted
	peanuts, home roasted
salted	unsalted
peanut butter w/sugar,	peanut butter, peanuts only,
partially hydrogenated fat	salted or unsalted
SALT	SALT (p. 31)
table salt	unrefined mineral salt
	sea salt
MISC.	MISC. (pp.41-42)
chocolate, sweetened	unsweetened chocolate
	cocoa powder
	low fat cocoa powder
cocoa powder	low-fat cocoa powder
	carob powder
chocolate chips	carob chips, unsweetened
coconut, sweetened	unsweetened coconut

Every prudent man acts out of knowledge. . . Proverbs 13:16

How to Turn Favorite Desserts
into Nutritional Pluses

~ Use whole wheat flour (preferrably whole wheat pastry flour for lightness) in place of white flour. For a transition step, use half whole wheat flour and half unbleached white flour. See pp. 20-22.

~ In cakes replace ¼ of the flour with arrowroot powder for a lighter, finer texture.

~ Use honey or crystalline fructose in place of sugar, using half as much, or use *Sucanat* (p. 26) in same amount. A combination of these may also be used. See pp. 26-29.

~ Use unsalted butter or canola oil in place of shortening or margarine. Salted butter may be used, but it adds unnecessary sodium. Olive oil can be used in most cakes without the flavor coming through. See pp. 32-33.

~ Reduce the amount of fat called for to half the amount. To omit fat from recipes, see pp. 33-34.

~ Reduce the amount of nuts called for by half.

~ Reduce the salt by half; use a quality sea salt or mineral salt. Adjust amount up or down according to taste. See p. 31.

~ Use a cultured milk in place of milk, such as buttermilk, sour milk, or yogurt; use lowfat or nonfat. See p. 39.

~ Use 2 egg whites in place of each egg, if desired. Other alternatives are also available. See p. 39.

~ Use carob in place of all or half the chocolate or use low-fat, decaffeinated cocoa powder. Use unsweetened carob chips in place of chocolate chips, if desired. Reduce chocolate chips to half the amount. See pp. 41-42.

~ Use the chart, *Choosing Ingredient Alternatives*, pp. 9-11, to substitute other more nutritious ingredients. Make one change in a recipe at a time in order to trace results to specific changes.

~ If substitutions significantly change the original consistency of the dough or batter, increase or decrease dry ingredients or liquids accordingly to achieve about the same consistency.

Shopping for Ingredients

Ingredients used in **Desserts** or suggested for allergy alternatives are listed below. It is not necessary to stock your kitchen with every ingredient. Most items may be purchased at the supermarket or at a health food store. Other sources include mail order and food co-ops. A few sources for these and specialty items that may not be locally available are listed on pp. 16-18.

<u>Available at Health Food Stores</u> *(see page numbers for more information)*

almonds, unroasted, unsalted--better price than supermarkets
apples, dried, unsulfured *(p. 40)*
apricots, dried, unsulfured *(p. 40)*
arrowroot powder--better price than supermarkets *(pp. 19, 44)*
baking powder, low sodium *(p. 44)*
baking powder, *Rumford*; also at some supermarkets *(p. 44)*
barley, hulled whole, flour and/or grain *(pp. 16, 20)*
brewer's yeast *(for recipe, p. 89, only)*
brown rice, flour and/or grain *(p. 20)*
brown rice cereal, crispy whole *(p. 22; for recipe, p. 110 only)*
buttermilk, powdered (e.g *Darigold*) *(p. 39)*
butter, unsalted, certified raw (limited availability) *(pp. 17, 32)*
canola oil (e.g *Spectrum Naturals, Arrowhead Mills*) *(p. 32)*
carob chips, unsweetened (e.g *Sunspire*) *(p. 42)*
carob powder, toasted; also at many supermarkets *(p. 41)*
cocoa powder, low-fat (e.g *WonderSlim*) *(pp. 18, 42)*
coconut, unsweetened *(p. 42)*
crystalline fructose *(pp. 16, 27)*
date dices or nuggets, *(pp. 16, 40)*
date sugar *(p. 29)*
dried apples, unsulfured *(pp. 16, 40, 111, 136)*
dried fruits, unsulfured *(p. 40)*
eggs, fertile or range fed *(pp. 18, 39)*
fat & egg substitutes (e.g *WonderSlim, Just like Shortenin'*) *(pp. 18)*
flax seeds *(p. 16; for recipe, p. 103, only)*
flours, nut (e.g *Omega Nutrition*) *(pp. 17, 22)*
flours/grains, whole grain *(pp. 16, 19)*
fruit spreads, honey-sweetened, all-fruit or 100% fruit (also at supermarkets) *(p. 41)*
graham crackers, whole grain (e.g *Mi-Del, New Morning*) *(p. 22)*
honey, unheated *(p. 24)*
Kamut, flour, grain, cereal flakes *(pp. 16, 21)*
kefir, fruit flavors, pasteurized, certified raw (e.g *Steuve's Natural*--availability limited) *(pp. 18, 39)*

lecithin granules *(for recipe, p. 89, only)*

mayonnaise, no refined sugars or preservatives (e.g *Hain)* *(p. 70)*

molasses, blackstrap or dark, unsulfured *(p. 27)*

millet *(for recipe, p. 146, only)*

millet, puffed cereal *(pp. 22, for recipe, p. 104 only)*

Mystic Lake Dairy Mixed Fruit Concentrate Sweetener *(pp. 17, 28)*

nonfat dry milk powder, non-instant *(p. 39)*

nuts (most), unroasted, unsalted *(p. 43)*

oat bran; also at supermarkets *(pp. 20-21)*

oats, rolled; also at supermarkets

olive oil, virgin (e.g *Spectrum Naturals, Arrowhead Mills)* *(pp. 16, 32)*

olive oil non-stick spray; also at many supermarkets *(p. 54)*

pecans--often better price than supermarket *(p. 43)*

protein powder *(for recipes, pp. 103, 111, only)*

rice milk (e.g. *Rice Dream Non-Dairy Beverage)* *(p. 39)*

salt (e.g. *RealSalt)* *(pp. 18, 31)*

sesame seeds, unroasted, unsalted *(p. 43)*

soy milk or tofu beverage (e.g. *Better Than Milk)* *(p. 39)*

spelt, flour and/or grain *(pp. 16, 20)*

sunflower seeds *(for recipe, p. 43, only)*

Sucanat, whole cane sugar *(p. 26)*

tapioca, small pearl *(for recipe, p. 147, only)*

tofu (organic), soft or regular *(for recipe, p. 112, only)*

vanilla extract, without added sugar (e.g. *Cook's Choice)* *(p.43)*

whipping cream, certified raw--availability limited *(p. 17)*

whole wheat pastry flour *(pp. 16, 19)*

yogurt, with active cultures; plain, vanilla; lowfat, nonfat *(p. 39)*

yogurt, pasteurized, not homogenized (e.g. *Brown Cow)* *(pp. 18, 39)*

Available at Supermarkets

almonds (usually better price at health food stores) *(p. 43)*

all-fruit or 100% spreads (no sugar) *(p. 41)*

almond extract

applesauce, unsweetened

apricot nectar (canned fruit juices) *(for recipe, p. 144, only)*

baking powder, *Rumford* (limited) *(p.44)*

baking soda

brown rice, long grain *(pp. 20-21)*

buttermilk, ½%, 1%, 1½%, 2% fat *(p. 39)*

buttermilk, cultured powder (e.g. *Seco)*--limited availability *(p. 39)*

butter, unsalted *(p. 32)*

canola oil *(p. 32)*

carob powder *(p. 41)*

    chocolate chips, unsweetened

    chocolate, unsweetened--squares, cocoa powder *(p. 41)*

    cornstarch *(p. 44)*

    cream cheese, light or *Neufchatel*, soft, regular

    cream of tartar (spice shelf)

    dates, pitted

    eggs, battery (from caged, non-range fed chickens) *(p. 39)*

    egg substitute (e.g. *Egg Beaters*) *(p. 39)*

    extracts, almond, coconut, orange, lemon, mint, vanilla, etc.

    figs, dried black (e.g. *Black Mission*)

    fruits, canned unsweetened

    fruits, frozen unsweetened

    gelatine, unflavored (e.g. *Knox*) *(p. 44)*

    grapefruit juice, canned unsweetened *(for recipe, p. 144, only)*

    honey (uncooked is best but limited in availability) *(p. 24)*

    honey, spun *(for recipe, p. 65, only)*

    lemon juice, bottled (but fresh lemon juice preferred)

    lemon peel, dried (spice shelf)

    molasses, light or mild, dark; unsulfured *(p. 27)*

    oat bran *(pp. 20-21)*

    olive oil *(p. 32)*

    olive oil non-stick spray (e.g. *Pam*) *(p. 54)*

    orange peel, dried (spice shelf)

    raisins

    ricotta cheese, skim milk *(for recipe, p. 85, only)*

    rolled oats, quick and old-fashioned (e.g *Quaker*)

    peanut butter, peanuts, salt only (e.g *Laura Scudder's*) *(p. 43)*

    pecans--often better price at health food stores *(p. 43)*

    persimmons, in season--limited availability *(pp. 108, 126, 140)*

    pineapple, unsweetened, fruit or juice

    poppy seeds (spice shelf) *(for recipe, p. 78, only)*

    pumpkin, canned *(pp. 98, 127)*

    sour cream, nonfat, light, regular (e.g *Knudsen, Sealtest*) *(p. 128)*

    spices (cinnamon, cloves, nutmeg, ginger, allspice, coriander)

    tapioca, instant or quick cooking *(p. 147)*

    tofu, soft or regular *(for recipes, pp. 112, 124, 125 only)*

    unflavored gelatine (e.g *Knox*) *(p. 44)*

    vanilla, pure

    walnuts

    wheat germ, toasted vacuum packed jar (e.g. *Kretchmer*)

    whipping cream, ultra-pasteurized *(p. 155)*

    yogurt, with active cultures; plain, vanilla; lowfat, nonfat *(p. 39)*

MAIL ORDER SOURCES

Write or call companies for current catalogue and full range of products. Only ingredients used in **Desserts** are listed here. Be aware that companies come and go, change locations, phone numbers, and product offerings.

JAFFE BROS. INC.
P.O. Box 636
Valley Center, CA 92082-0636
(619) 749-1133

Organic fruit jams made with honey; almonds; unsulfured dried apples; hulled whole grain barley; long grain brown rice; expeller pressed canola oil; carob powder; unsweetened coconut; dates; unsulfured Black Mission figs; flax seeds; unheated honey; Kamut flour or whole grain Kamut; lecithin granules; pure Vermont maple syrup; soy milk powder; oat groats; unprocessed extra virgin organic olive oil; unsalted organic peanut butter; peanuts; pecans; raisins; rolled oats; unrefined sea salt; spelt flour or whole grain spelt; sesame and sunflower seeds; soy; walnuts; whole wheat pastry flour or grain.

Wide organic selection. In business for 45 years
Mail Order; UPS Shipping nationwide
Phone order with Visa or MasterCard accepted

WALNUT ACRES ORGANIC FARMS
Penns Creek, PA 17862
Toll free order line: 1-800-433-3998
Discovery, Visa, MasterCard accepted
Fax: 1-717-837-1146
24-Hour order service
Second day or overnight delivery available
Full color catalogue available

Granolas and cereals, whole grain flours, whole grains, nuts, seeds, dried fruits, raisins, fresh produce, canned unsweetened fruits, honey or juice-sweetened jams, peanut butter, nut butters, arrowroot powder, nonfat dry milk powder, buttermilk powder, powdered soy milk, maple syrup, rice syrup, *Sucanat*, sorghum syrup, honey, low sodium baking powder, wheat germ, oat bran, real vanilla, stainless steel bakeware, grain mills, cocoa, extra virgin olive oil, canola oil, cookies, gift items.

BOB'S RED MILL NATURAL FOODS, INC.
5209 S.E. International Way
Milwaukie, OR 97222
(503) 654-3215   fax (503) 653-1339
UPS Shipping   VISA and MasterCard accepted

Dried apples, arrowroot, barley, barley flour, carob, date pieces, date sugar, granolas, brown rice, brown rice flour, buttermilk powder, fructose, lecithin granules, nonfat dry milk powder, millet, millet flour, oat bran, oats, poppy, sesame, and sunflower seeds, raisins, sea salt, spelt, spelt flour, tapioca, pastry grain, whole wheat pastry flour, wheat germ

SPECIALTY ITEM SOURCES

***Mystic Lake Dairy* Mixed Fruit Concentrate Sweetener** *(p. 28)*
Mystic Lake Dairy
1439 244th Avenue N.E.
Redmond, WA 99053
(206) 868-2029

Natural sweetener recipe book also available.

***Omega Nutrition* Nut Flours** (gluten-free) *(p. 22)*
Omega Nutrition U.S.A., Inc.
6505 Aldrich Road
Bellingham, WA 98226
(800) 661-3529

Almond Flour, hazelnut flour, pistachio flour.

Request recipe information

Stainless Steel Waterless Cookware *(p. 47)*
Saladmaster Showroom
P.O. Box 27114
Tampa, Florida 33688
Robert J. (Jack) Eley, President (813) 961-5877

***Steuve's Natural* Raw Certified Dairy Products** *(p. 39)*
AltaDena Dairies, Some Health Food Stores
Limited primarily to California

Cheddar cheese; butter; fertile (range fed) eggs;
kefir; milk; whipping cream.

Eggs, Range Fed or Fertile
AltaDena Dairies, California
Trader Joe Markets, Southern California
Fresh Eggs sold by local farmers in many states

RealSalt Unrefined Mineral Salt *(p. 31)*
American Orsa, Inc.
75 No. State
Redmond, Utah 84652
(801) 529-7487

Price and product list available.
1 lb, 2 lb, 5 lb, 25 lb, 50 lb sizes available
Request free literature with your order
Phone order with Visa or MasterCard accepted

WonderSlim Low-Fat Cocoa Powder *(p. 42)*
WonderSlim Fat & Egg Substitute *(p. 33)*
Natural Food Technologies, Inc
P.O. Box 1436
Montebello, CA 90640
(800) 497-6595

For free cooking recipes send self-addressed, stamped envelope to:
WonderSlim, P.O. Box 1436, Montebello, CA 90640

Just like Shortenin' (fruit concentrate fat substitute) *(p. 33)*
The PlumLife Comany, Inc.
15 Orchard Park
Madison, CT 06443
(203) 245-5993

Yogurt, Pasteurized (not homogenized) *(p. 39)*
Trader Joe's Cream Line Yogurt, Plain
Trader Joe Markets, Southern California.

She is like the merchant ships,
bringing her food from afar.
Proverbs 31:14

About Flours & Grains

. . .the valleys are mantled with grain,
they shout for joy and sing. Psalm 65:13

Whole grains as used in desserts is briefly discussed below. For more complete information see **Breakfasts** (pp. 45-86).

Whole Wheat Pastry Flour

Whole wheat pastry flour is my first alternative choice for white flour in most dessert recipes. Pastry flour usually comes from soft spring wheat, a different variety of wheat than bread flour. Because it is lower in gluten content than bread flour, whole wheat pastry flour produces lighter cakes, cookies, and other desserts made without yeast. However, bread flour, primarily from hard winter red wheat, can be used in dessert recipes. It is my first preference for pie crusts (p. 115). Bread flour, labeled *Whole Wheat Flour* or *100% Whole Wheat Flour*, is the kind of whole wheat flour usually available in supermarkets. For whole wheat pastry flour or grain, check out health food stores and mail order sources (pp. 14, 16, 17).

Unbleached White Flour

White flour is not recommended in **Desserts** except as an option in *Coconut Macaroons*, p. 94, and *Joy's 4-in-1 Non-Dairy Sauce*, p. 159. Unbleached white flour is a step better nutritionally, but it is still devoid of most of the original nutrients and most of the dietary fiber (*See* comparison chart, **Breakfasts,** p. 52, or **Lunches & Snacks**, p. 106). Enrichment of white flour by synthetically increasing the content of three B-vitamins and iron does not restore either the original nutritional balance or the fiber. Nevertheless, if you find the transition from white flour to entirely whole grain flour too radical, start with half unbleached white flour and half whole wheat pastry flour. Most supermarkets carry unbleached white flour. If the package does not designate "unbleached" assume it is bleached.

Alternatives to Wheat Flour   See pp. 20-22.

Arrowroot or Cornstarch to Lighten Cakes

Arrowroot is a starch that comes from the tubers of several tropical plants. It contains trace minerals and is therefore a more complete food than cornstarch. To lighten cakes, ¼ the flour may be replaced with an equal amount of arrowroot powder or cornstarch. Arrowroot powder may be purchased more economically in larger packages at health food stores than at supermarkets.

FLOUR ALTERNATIVES FOR WHEAT FLOUR

Cakes: 2 parts barley flour with 1 part long grain brown rice flour works well (e.g. 2 cups barley flour to 1 cup brown rice flour). I have tested this combination successfully in *Applesauce Cake* (p. 66), *Gingerbread Cake* (p. 74), and *Brownies* (p. 88). It will work in most other cake recipes, as well. Barley flour is also often satisfactory used alone for cakes.

Cookies: a blend of barley flour, long grain brown rice flour, and optional oat bran works well in place of whole wheat pastry flour. I have tested this blend in *Date Walnut Cookies* (p. 96), *Hobo Fortune Cookies* (p. 101), *Orange or Lemon Spice Cookies* (p. 106), and *Chocolate Drop Cookies* (p. 92), It will work in the other cookie recipes, as well. The texture and flavor are pleasing, although the cookies tend to spread a bit more. Use barley flour milled from hulled whole barley, not pearled barley, to get full nutritional value. To purchase, see pp. 13, 16, 17.

The ratio of flours for cookies is approximately 4 parts barley flour, 2 parts brown rice flour, and 1 part oat bran flour (e.g. 1 cup barley flour + ½ cup brown rice flour + ¼ cup oat bran). Use this as a reference point for altering other recipes you may want to change. In the chart on p. 21 I have modified this ratio for convenient measuring for any cookie recipe found in **Desserts**.

There are 2 ways to preblend these grains for convenience:

1) **Flour Blend** Use this method if you do not have access to a grain mill. Blend together evenly: **8 cups barley flour** with **4 cups brown rice flour**; blend in **2 cups oat bran, optional.** Refrigerate in a tightly covered container. When making cakes or cupcakes, bring flour to room temperature.

2) **Pre-mixed grain** Use this method if you have a grain mill. Mix together **8 cups whole hulled barley** with **4 cups long grain brown rice**. Mill the required amount of grain mix to produce the amount of barley + brown rice flour called for in recipe just before making it. Add oat bran, if desired, at that time.

For grain measurements needed for milling the desired amount of flour, consult **Breakfasts**, *Grain to Flour Conversion Chart*, p. 85. As a general rule of thumb, 1 cup grain will produce about 1½ cups flour, but always measure the flour after milling the grain.

Flour Amounts to Replace
Wheat Flour in Cookies

For ¼ C. wheat flour use:
2½ Tbsps. barley flour
1½ Tbsps. brown rice flour

For ½ C. wheat flour use:
5 Tbsps. barley flour
3 Tbsps. brown rice flour

For ¾ C. wheat flour use:
½ cup barley flour
¼ cup brown rice flour

For 1 C. wheat flour use:
2/3 cup barley flour
1/3 cup brown rice flour

For 1¼ C. wheat flour use:
¾ cup barley flour
6 Tbsps. brown rice flour
2 Tbsps. oat bran

For 1½ C. wheat flour use:
1 cup barley flour
½ cup brown rice flour

For 1 2/3 C. wheat flour use:
1 1/8 cups barley flour
½ cup brown rice flour
optional: 1/8 cup oat bran
in place of 1/8 cup barley flour

For 1¾ C. wheat flour use:
1 cup barley flour
½ cup brown rice flour
¼ cup oat bran

For 2 C. wheat flour use:
1¼ cups barley flour
½ cup brown rice flour
¼ cup oat bran

For 2½ - 2 5/8 C. wheat flour use:
1½ cups barley flour
¾ cup brown rice flour
¼ - 3/8 cup (6 Tbsps.) oat bran

For 3 C. wheat flour use:
1¾ cups barley flour
7/8 cup brown rice flour
(¾ cup + 2 Tbsps.)
3/8 cup oat bran (6 Tbsps.)

For 3¼ C. wheat flour use:
2 cups barley flour
1 cup brown rice flour
¼ cup oat bran

Other Flours to Replace Wheat Flour

Both Kamut and spelt work well in place of whole wheat pastry flour in most **Dessert** recipes. Although both are wheat varieties, many people allergic to common wheats can handle Kamut and/ or spelt. Use Kamut flour in same amount as wheat flour in recipes. Use a little more spelt, about 1/3 - 2/3 cup more, or as needed in a recipe to achieve the same consistency in the dough. I have tested these grains successfully in many waffle, pancake, muffin, coffeecake, and crepe recipes, and in several cookie recipes. Try the delicious *Kamut-Oatmeal* and *Kamut-Flake Cookies*, p. 102. For more information about these grains see **Breakfasts**, pp. 61-64.

Nut Flours

Nut flours offer gluten-free alternatives for grain flours in dessert recipes. Request availability and recipe information from *Omega Nutrition* (see p. 17). Observe from the recipe information how nut flour is used in recipes. This information may then be adapted to recipes in **Desserts**.

Buying & Storing Flours & Grains

For purchasing grains and flours, see pp 13-17. Grains are often more readily available than flours, store longer, contain more long-lasting nutrient value, and produce lighter and fresher tasting recipes. To use grains you need a grain mill (see **Breakfasts**, p. 84). Store flours, brans, and wheat germ in refrigerator or freezer (preferred if there is room) and grains in a cool, dry place (see **Breakfasts**, p. 80-81). Bring flour to room temperature before using for best results in cakes or cupcakes.

Arrowroot or cornstarch may be stored at room temperature.

Graham Crackers

For graham cracker crusts and toppings I use *Mi-Del* or *New Morning Honey Grahams* from the health food store. Not all brands of whole grain graham crackers are as tasty as these two. Compare the ingredients used in *Mi-Del Honey Grahams* (100% Whole Wheat) with a typical supermarket brand, p. 6.

Whole grain crackers containing no preservatives will go rancid quickly. It is therefore important to store them in the freezer or at least in the refrigerator unless planning to use them up in a couple of weeks. However, since each box will make about 4 graham cracker crusts, it isn't likely you'll use them all right away. Store them in the original box. Store any leftover opened cracker packages or crushed crackers in a freezer ziploc bag.

Whole Grain Breakfast Cereals

For that yummy favorite rice crispy cookie recipe, you'll find crispy brown rice cereal made from whole grain brown rice in health food stores, such as *Grainfield's* brand. In fact, for any cookie recipe calling for a breakfast cereal, the whole grain alternative is undoubtedly available at a health food store. Like whole grain crackers, these do not contain preservatives. Store them in the freezer if you are not using them right away and seal opened cereal in a freezer ziploc bag.

About Sugars

Perhaps you've heard that the latest research studies indicate that sugar does not cause hyperactivity in children (empty calories, tooth decay, and other negative effects of sugar notwithstanding). Parents, whose children are still climbing the walls after sugar treats, are reacting with varying degrees of skepticism, alarm, and frustration.

Jean Carper in *The Food Pharmacy* (Bantam Books, July, 1988, pp. 284-288) explains in a fairly understandable way how the studies seem to contradict parents' observations.

To summarize Jean Carper: Sugar triggers the release of insulin in the blood stream that triggers the chemical tryptophan which produces the brain chemical, serotonin. Serotonin is a neurotransmitter that has a calming effect "'As a result, you feel less stressed, less anxious, more focused and relaxed.' says Dr. Judith Wurtman, leading MIT researcher on the subject." (p. 285). Research even shows that about 2½ tablespoons (30 grams) sugar produces this result, and that more neither decreases or increases this effect (**sugar ☞ insulin ☞ tryptophan ☞ serotonin ☞ calming effect**). And Carper actually goes on with more good things to say. So let's head for the desserts!? Wait! There are a few cautions:

~ Protein and fat slow down this "wonder effect" of sugar. Therefore, don't expect quite so dramatic a result from the dessert habit (anyone for no-fat, no-egg, no-dairy dessert?).

~ Fruit sugars don't produce the same effect--so much for fructose, fruits, and fruit concentrates as sugar substitutes for this effect.

~ Sugar still contributes to cavities--even calcium, iron, and potassium-rich blackstrap molasses.

~ Some persons' consumption of a little sugar "drives" them to eat more sugar (too much more?), i.e. it can be addictive.

~ Refined sugars have virtually no nutrient value (empty calories).

~ Sugar combined with starch in dessert often causes digestive stress and distress, especially for older adults.

~ If you don't sleep well, eat 3 *"Fat Free"* Oatmeal Cookies, p. 91, before you go to bed. Sounds good! Think I'll try it. I don't think I've been sleeping so well lately.

Much has been researched and written on the effects of sugar, especially refined sugar, on the human body. Not the least of these is that the digestion of all sugars robs the body of nutrients, particularly B-vitamins and chromium--again, especially true of sugars that contain no nutritional value. Whenever the body is robbed of nutrients the door of opportunity to a host of health problems is opened. I follow these guiding principles in the use of sugars:

1. Choose sugars that are as near as possible to containing their original full range of nutrients.

2. Use them in strict moderation (i.e. making desserts the occasional treat instead of a part of the daily menu).

3. Use other ingredients in dessert recipes that are nutrient-rich--especially using whole grain flours that are high in dietary fiber and the B-vitamins.

Reread the second caution, p. 23, about fruit sugars not producing the calming effect of other sugars. This in no way suggests that fresh fruits are not our very best desserts. In fact, I call them God's desserts. Raw fresh fruits still contain all their wonderful health-promoting enzymes. Secondly, they contain a range of vitamins and minerals packaged in a natural high-fiber medium that enables the body to digest and metabolize them more effectively. And because they are a whole food, many other health-giving properties that we hardly yet understand are also included. Try *Orange Ambrosia* or *Elegant Fruit Platter*, pp. 138, 142. Why not eat a piece of fresh fruit, out-of-hand, for dessert? No preparation, no utensils, no baking!

Honey

> *Eat honey, my son, for it is good; honey from the comb is sweet to your taste. . . If you find honey, eat just enough--too much of it, and you will vomit. Proverbs 24:13; 25:16*

Some nutritional purists and traditionalists tend to give honey mixed reviews. I believe further study will substantiate that what is recorded in the Bible is true. *It is the glory of God to conceal a matter; to search out a matter is the glory of kings. Proverbs 25:2.* We do know that honey contains an incredibly wide range of minute amounts of nutrients. The fact that these nutritients are in minute amounts does not mean they are not valuable. Frances Sheridan Goulart says in *Sugar Substitutes, The Herbalist, November*, 1979, pp. 21-22:

> Containing 39 percent fructose, honey is an important anti-fatigue food. Since it is predigested, it builds up the alkaline reserves in the blood and tissues, and provides maximum energy with a minimum of shock to the digestive system. In addition to protein from the pollen (the substance responsible for clouding in unfiltered honey), good honey contains some vitamin A, several vitamins from the B complex, and vital enzymes and minerals such as phosphorus, potassium, calcium, sodium, sulphur, iron, magnesium, and manganese--all in the right small amounts and balance to serve the needs of the normal individual.

The proverbial meaning of eating honey *from the comb* is not clear, but may suggest the importance of purchasing honey as unprocessessed as possible for minimal nutrient destruction. I do suggest that *unfiltered, unheated* honey is the best quality choice. It is admittedly more expensive and normally available only in health food stores or from local bee keepers. It can often be purchased in bulk, as in 60 lb. plastic buckets, at a savings. In cooking, I prefer to minimize the heating of honey to a high temperature over direct heat. Thus, you won't find too many *Almond Roca* (p. 83) type recipes in **Desserts.**

Eat just enough. When my family made the transition from white refined sugar to honey, we also considerably reduced the frequency of desserts. In addition, because honey is significantly sweeter than sugar, one may normally use half as much as white sugar. 1 cup white sugar contains 768 calories and 192 grams carbohydrate compared to ½ cup honey containing 516 calories and 138 grams carbohydrate.

My children have become accustomed now to the deeper-richer flavor of baked products with honey rather than the intensely sweet flavor of white sugar. But if too much honey is used, the flavor is too dominating. Honey is the product of many different flower nectars, flavors range from mild to strong. Lighter honeys are generally milder flavored, darker honeys stronger. In baking the difference is not as noticable as in puddings or milk-based desserts. Sometimes stronger flavored honey is sold in bulk as "Baker's Honey." It is often less expensive. Tupelo honey is known to be especially acceptable for diabetics.

Big pluses for using honey are its wide availability and relatively low cost compared to other natural sugars (see p. 30).

Cane or Beet Sugar

White sugar is 99.9% nutrient-free. What about the lesser refined cane sugars, such as raw sugar, Turbinado sugar, and brown sugar? Raw sugar and Turbinado sugar are typically available in health food stores. Both are brown in appearance and refined, containing more of the original nutrients than white sugar. Turbinado sugar contains less original nutrients than raw sugar. Brown sugar, too, is certainly a better choice than white sugar, but none of these have the nutritional benefit of the whole sugar cane juice.

Until recently whole sugar cane was not available in the U.S.A. in a conveniently usable form. Now, however, an excellent whole cane sugar called *Sucanat* (an abbreviation of SUgar CAne NATural) is being marketed in health food stores. *Sucanat* is evaporated whole sugar cane juice, containing its full range of nutrients. Note the comparison in nutrient content with white refined sugar and brown sugar:

1 CUP (150 gm)	*SUCANAT**	BROWN SUGAR*	WHITE SUGAR *
Calories	570	541**	768
Carbohydrate	144 mg	140 gm**	192 gm
Vit. A	1600 IU	0	0
Vit. C	49.5 mg	0	0
Vit. B-1	0.21 mg	0.01 mg	0
Vit. B-2	0.21 mg	0.04 mg	0
Vit. B-3	0.20 mg	0.20 mg	0
Vit. B-6	0.60 mg	0.30 mg	0
Calcium	165 mg	127 mg	0
Iron	6.5 mg	5 mg	0.20 mg
Potassium	11125 mg	514 mg	4.5 mg

*nutrient data taken from *Sucanat* can label.
**nutrient data taken from other sources (see p. 59)

Sucanat also contains phosphorus, magnesium, zinc, copper, pantothenic acid, and chromium.

I have been delighted with the results of *Sucanat* in baking. It is a good alternative for honey, giving variation in flavor and texture. It has restored some of the desired crispiness in cookies while honey and fructose produce cookies that are cake-like in texture. Use the same amount of *Sucanat* as white or brown sugar or twice as much as honey for most recipes.

Fructose

Fructose is available in both liquid and crystalline form. Crystalline fructose is a white granular sugar identical in appearance to white sugar. It is also known as levulose or fruit sugar. The form of sugar in cane or beet sugar, on the other hand, is sucrose. Crystalline fructose is most often derived from corn. While it is highly refined with almost no nutritional value, it has two advantages over refined cane or beet sugar: 1) Fructose causes less release of insulin in the blood stream, an advantage for diabetics and hypoglycemics 2) Though not twice as sweet as white sugar, ½ the amount typically works well in most recipes, reducing calories and grams of sugar.

Before *Sucanat* became available, I used crystalline fructose more frequently. I still use it occasionally as in *Angel Food Cake*, p. 68, *Orange Chiffon Cake*, p. 75, and in puddings. Crystalline fructose can be used interchangeably with honey in the same amount in any recipe.

Most health food stores carry fructose. I usually purchase it in a 5 lb. bag, which lasts quite a while. Store it in a tightly covered container to prevent exposure to moisture. If moisture gets inside, it will become hard as rock.

Molasses

A by-product in the processing of cane or beet sugar, molasses, especially *blackstrap* (usually only available at health food stores), contains a goldmine of the nutrients extracted from refined white sugar. It is a good source of B-vitamins and an excellent source of calcium, iron, and potassium. Generally two types are available in supermarkets: *light* or *mild* molasses, what remains after the first extraction in the processing of white sugar, and *dark* or *medium*, what remains after the second extraction. *Blackstrap* molasses is what remains after the third extraction. The following table shows the differences in nutritional values:

1 Cup Molasses	Blackstrap	Dark (Medium)	Light (Mild)
Calories	699	761	827
Carbohydrate	180 mg	299 gm	210 mg
Vit. B-1	.36 mg	NA	.23 mg
Vit. B-2	.62 mg	.39 mg	0.2 mg
Vit. B-3	6.6 mg	3.9 mg	0.7 mg
Vit. B-6	.67 mg	.67 mg	.66 mg
Calcium	2200 mg	950 mg	340 mg
Iron	53 mg	20 mg	14 mg
Potassium	9600 mg	3500 mg	3000 mg

I usually use blackstrap molasses even though the flavor is considerably stronger than light or dark molasses. Molasses flavor, in general, does not blend as well in most dessert recipes as in muffins or breads. To experiment with molasses, substitute ¼ of the sweetening in the recipe with molasses, beginning with the strength of flavor (mild, medium, or blackstrap) that you prefer. Purchase molasses that is *unsulfured*. This should be stated on the jar. Store it in a cupboard. It will last indefinitely.

Molasses also has a laxative effect which may be too strong for some people, but very helpful to others.

Fruit Concentrates

Several different types of fruit concentrates can be used as sweeteners in dessert recipes: frozen unsweetened fruit juice concentrate, all fruit spread (jam), or a concentrated fruit sweetener in liquid form such as *Cascadian Farms* Organic Fruit Sweetener (White Grape Juice Concentrate) or *Mystic Lake Dairy Sweetener Mixed Fruit Concentrate* (100% pineapple syrup, pear and peach juice concentrate). For information and availability of *Mystic Lake Dairy Sweetener Mixed Fruit Concentrate*, see p. 17.

Nutrient information for these may be very limited or not available, but it may be assumed to be higher than that of crystalline fructose. As fruit sugars they may have the same effect on insulin release into the blood stream (see fructose, p. 27).

Mystic Lake Dairy Sweetener Mixed Fruit Concentrate works well in in *"Fat Free" Oatmeal Cookies*, p. 91. Most fruit concentrates of syrupy consistency such as *Mystic Lake* and *Cascadian Farms* may be expected to work similarly in recipes. All-fruit jam or frozen juice concentrates will work somewhat differently in strength of sweetness and resulting texture.

To experiment with substitution, begin by substituting 1 cup fruit concentrate for 1 cup other sweetener, or for ½ cup fructose or honey. Reduce other liquid or increase flour accordingly to keep batter or dough consistency the same (see p. 33). After you have taste-tested an experimental recipe, adjust the sweetening to taste.

New fruit sources are also being manufactured for use as fat or fat and egg substitutes, as *Just like Shortenin'* and *WonderSlim Fat & Egg Substitute* (see p. 33). Use of these may reduce the amount of sweetening needed in some recipes.

FruitSource

FruitSource, an all-purpose liquid or granular sweetener made from grapes and brown rice is a recent arrival in health food stores. Granular *FruitSource* works well in *"Fat Free" Oatmeal Cookies*, p. 91, substituting 1 cup for 1 cup other sweetener, or 1 cup in place of ½ cup fructose or honey.

Other Sweeteners

There are certainly other sweeteners available, primarily in health foods stores, such as date sugar, rice syrup, sorghum syrup, barley malt syrup, maple syrup, maple sugar, dextrose, etc. Except for occasional use of date sugar (as in *Date Sugar Cookies*, p. 86), I do not use these sweeteners in dessert recipes. To use date sugar substitute 1 cup packed date sugar for 1 cup packed brown sugar or 1 cup *Sucanat*.

Stevia Rebaudiana Extract is an herb product to use in low sugar cooking and baking, available in health food stores. For resource information on this product see **Breakfasts**, p. 15.

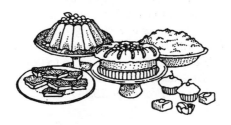

29

Comparing Costs of Sweeteners

Unfamiliarity, availablity, and expense are probably the main obstacles to more wholesome sweeteners. After all, when a cup of white sugar costs only $.19 per cup and a cup of brown sugar only $.28 per cup, it may seem difficult to justify a more expensive alternative. The chart below compares the 1995-96 prices of some of the available sweeteners (prices rise, on the average, about 3% per year). This comparison is based on the approximate equivalent amounts that normally are used in recipes (e.g. 1 cup white sugar, brown sugar, *Sucanat* or fruit concentrate as equivalent to ½ cup honey or ½ cup crystalline fructose):

1 cup white cane or beet sugar	$ .19
1 cup brown sugar	$ .28
½ cup crystaline fructose	$ .28
½ cup honey	$ .47
1 cup *Sucanat*	$1.08
1 cup date sugar	$1.56
1 cup *FruitSource*, granular	$1.86
1 cup real maple syrup	$1.95
1 cup *Mystic Lake Dairy Mixed Fruit Concentrate*	$2.80

The alternative sweeteners seem very expensive, but check out some of the comparative costs of cookies made with them, pp. 90-91--from $.06 to $.12 per cookie. You can hardly buy cookies with homebaked goodness in that price range.

Do not eat the food of a stingy man,
do not crave his delicacies,
for he is the kind of man
who is always thinking about the cost.
"Eat and drink," he says to you
but his heart is not with you.
Proverbs 23:6-7

About Salt

Americans, on the average, consume 2 to 3 times as much sodium as the USDA recommended limit of 1100 to 3300 mg. You don't have to eliminate salt from recipes to maintain this recommended limit. Some nutritionists preach that once your taste buds adjust, food tastes wonderful without salt. I am skeptical about their ability to judge taste. A little salt consistently adds a very subtle, but real, certain something to the flavor of many recipes. For example in making *Almond Roca*, p. 83, there is a slight, but distinct improvement in the flavor using lightly salted over unsalted butter. Usually whether butter is salted or unsalted makes little taste difference in most recipes. In this recipe it does. In many dessert recipes, salt subtly moderates the highly sweet flavor to a more pleasant sweetness.

To improve the nutritional quality when using salt, most our recipes contain less salt than originally. When experimenting with a recipe for the first time, I usually cut the salt called for in half, adjusting the amount after the first taste test for the next trial.

In addition to cutting the amount of salt in recipes, I recommend using a salt that has not been dried at high temperatures such as kiln-drying, which destroys the trace minerals. Look for salt that has been "sun -evaporated only," or unheated in processing. There are usually several brands of such salt in health food stores. I especially recommend *RealSalt*, a mined inland salt available in some health food stores and by mail order (see p. 18). In April, 1985 I purchased 96 lbs. of *RealSalt* by mail order. This supply lasted until February, 1994. For almost 9 years this salt cost my family $.26 per month! I reordered in March, 1994 and although the price had increased to about $.60 per month, it is still an inexpensive ingredient and should last well into the 21st century.

Jesus, used salt to illustrate a spiritual truth. *Salt is good, but if it loses its saltiness, how can it be made salty again? It is fit neither for the soil nor for the manure pile; it is thrown out (Luke 14:34).* Blah food and blah people both need a little salt to spark interest.

 *Let your conversation be always full of grace,
seasoned with salt, so that you may know
how to answer everyone.
Colossians 4:6*

About Fats

Butter gives the best flavor of all the fats, and is a better nutritional choice than hydrogenated fats such as margarine or shortening (see *Breakfasts*, p. 264).

I prefer unsalted butter in baking for the purpose of reducing the sodium. Seldom have I noticed any difference in the flavor of any dessert except in *Almond Roca*, p. 83, and pie crusts. Lightly salted butter used in these recipes gives a subtle, but decidedly better flavor. Special care must be taken in the storage of unsalted butter. Since salt acts as a preservative, unsalted butter turns rancid much more quickly. The best place for it is in the freezer. For immediate use, it can be softened in the microwave at the simmering power level for a couple of minutes.

If desserts are served more frequently, I recommend using at least half oil in place of the butter in most dessert recipes, or experimenting with fat-free variations (see below). In baking I recommend use of a highly monounsaturated oil such as canola or olive oil rather than a more polyunsaturated oil such as safflower or soy oil (see *Main Dishes*, pp. 26-27 and *Breakfasts*, pp. 262-63). I am often asked if *Butter Spread* (*Breakfasts*, p. 265) can be used in baking. The answer is yes, but why use for baking what you troubled yourself to mix together for a spread? Just add oil and butter separately to the recipe. On the other hand, *Butter Spread* does provide a readily softened fat straight from the refrigerator.

If desired, oil may entirely replace butter. I prefer olive oil over canola oil if the flavor is not too strong. Even extra virgin olive oil works well in cakes. Unless a very light, mild olive oil is used, I recommend canola oil for cookies and pie crusts for more pleasing flavors.

I have often experimented by cutting the amount of butter in half without making any other changes in the other ingredients. The result is usually a pleasing but less rich flavor.

MAKING FAT FREE RECIPES

People are becoming much more conscious of fat. "Fat Free" has become an important part of the lablel on food products. Consequently, you'll want to know how to alter recipes in order to remove the fat. Should some other ingredient be added to replace the fat? New products are being developed to serve just this purpose (see *Fat and Egg Substitute Products*, pp. 33-34). Could the added fat be entirely eliminated? That challenge put me into my experimental cooking mode.

I made the recipe for *Chocolate or Carob Chip Cookies* with the oatmeal variation, p. 90, five times without the fat, keeping the other ingredients consistent, but varying only the type of sugar. The results were good as long as I adjusted the amount of the other ingredients to keep the dough at the original consistency. I discovered that when I used a granulated sweetener such as *Sucanat* (p. 26) or granular *FruitSource* (p. 29), leaving out the fat made a stiffer dough. To compensate, I added ¼ cup water. On the other hand, when I used a liquid sweetener* (except honey), such as *Mystic Lake Dairy Mixed Fruit Concentrate* (p. 28), leaving out the fat made a soupier dough. To compensate I added an extra ½ cup flour. This did not hold true when using honey because I used only half as much honey as the *Mystic Lake Dairy Mixed Fruit Concentrate*. To the recipe with honey, I actually added ¼ cup water to keep the consistency of the dough the same.

Four of the five fat free variations of *Chocolate or Carob Chip Cookies* tasted very good but varied slightly in texture from the original. Those made with honey lacked in pleasing sweetness, although freezing the cookies considerably improved the flavor. Perhaps increasing the honey by ¼ cup instead of adding the water might improve this variation as long as the honey is not too strong. Sugar flavors seemed to be more pronounced with the fat removed. The fat free doughs seemed to spread out a bit more than the original recipe if not chilled first. See the recipe for *"Fat Free" Oatmeal Cookies*, p. 91. To summarize a few guidelines:

~ Omit the fat from the recipe. Add water to the recipe to keep the original consistency if the recipe has honey or a granular sweetener* in it, such as *Sucanat*, granular *FruitSource*, brown sugar, or white sugar. In my experiment I found this to be ¼ cup water, but this could vary; aim at keeping the original consistency.

~ Omit the fat from the recipe. Add extra flour to the recipe to keep the original consistency if the recipe has a liquid sweetener* in it such as *Mystic Lake Dairy Mixed Fruit Concentrate*. In my experiment I found this to be about ½ cup flour, but this could vary; aim at keeping the original consistency.

*This does not apply to any liquid or granular artificial sweeteners.

Fat and Egg Substitute Products

I found two very new fat substitute products, *WonderSlim Fat & Egg Substitute* and *Just like Shortenin'*, at the Natural Products Expo in Anaheim, California. Both are used similarly in recipes to replace fat, and part or all, of the eggs. *WonderSlim* is made from water, dried plums, unbleached lecithin, and citric acid. *Just like Shortenin'* ingredients include dried plums, apples, and water. Virtually fat free, very low in sodium and containing no preservatives, both are advertised to make very moist baked goods. Half the amount of either one is used to replace the amount of fat called for in a recipe. For example, ¼ cup *Wonderslim* (35 calories) or ¼ cup *Just like Shortenin'* (168 calories) replaces ½ cup butter (1 stick), shortening, margarine, or oil (at over 800 calories). In cookies and brownies when *WonderSlim* is used to replace fat, 1½ teaspoons water can replace each egg. When using *Just like Shortenin'* to replace fat in a recipe, the eggs may be reduced by half. Because apples are one of the ingredients in *Just like Shortenin'*, it is a thicker and sweeter product than *WonderSlim*. Therefore, I would reduce the amount of sweetening called for in a recipe when using this product.

The cost of using these products is comparable to the cost of eggs and fat in recipes. Look for *Just like Shortenin'* and *WonderSlim* in health food stores. Eventually you will find them in some supermarkets. If you can't locate them, contact the source listed on pp. 17-18.

Recipe Fat Levels

Below is a list of the low fat, moderate fat, and high fat desserts in this book. The fat in many of these recipes could be further reduced by following the guidelines suggested above.

LOW FAT (30% OR LESS)

Cakes & Frostings

Honey Vanilla Frosting *(p. 69)*	0%
Angel Food Cake *(p. 63)*	1%
Applesauce Cupcakes, Honey Cream Frosting *(p. 64)*	16%
Applesauce Cupcakes, unfrosted *(p. 64)*	21%
Orange Chiffon Cake *(p. 75)*	21%
Honey Cream Frosting *(p. 65)*	21%
Poppy Seed Cake *(p. 78)*	27%
Gingerbread Cake *(p. 74)*	27%
Applesauce Cake, unfrosted *(p. 66)*	30%

Cookies

"Fat Free" Oatmeal Cookies *(p. 91)*	7%
Gingles *(p. 100)*	14%
Polynesian Squares, reduced fat *(p. 109)*	23%
Oatmeal Raisin Cookies *(p. 105)*	24%
Carob No-Bake Cookies *(p. 89)*	25%
Gingerbread People *(p. 99)*	30%

LOW FAT (30% OR LESS), CONT"D

Desserts

Rainbow Chiffon Jello Cubes *(p. 142)*	0%
Fruit Shrub *(p. 144)*	1%
Frozen Vanilla Yogurt *(p. 141)*	2%
Elegant Fruit Platter (Sample Fruit Platter for 8) *(p. 138-139)*	4%
Orange Ambrosia *(p. 142)*	18%
Persimmon Nut Bread *(p. 140)*	19%
Banana Nut Bread *(p. 140)*	20%
Baked Apples *(p. 132)*	27%
Fruit Cobbler *(p. 134)*	28%
Lemon Fruit Crepes *(p. 136)*	28%

Pies & Pie Crusts

Pumpkin Pie, reduced fat, single Rice Crust *(p. 127)*	21%
Fresh Apple Pie, single Rice Crust *(p. 120)*	26%
Fresh Berry Pie, single Rice Crust *(p. 120)*	27%
Carob Tofu Cheese Pie, Rice Crust *(p. 125)*	27%
Pumpkin Pie, Rice Crust *(p. 127)*	30%
Yogurt Pie *(p. 128)*	30%

Puddings & Custards

Tapioca, nonfat milk *(p. 147)*	
Apricot Yogurt Pudding *(p. 149)*	2%
Orange Yogurt Pudding *(p. 148)*	2%
Pineapple Yogurt Pudding *(p. 149)*	2%
Spiced Apple Yogurt Pudding *(p. 149)*	3%
Lite Chocolate Pudding *(p. 144)*	6%
Tapioca, lowfat milk *(p. 147)*	14%
Old Fashioned Rice Pudding *(p. 151)*	18%
Pineapple Kefir Pudding *(p. 150)*	18%
Vanilla Raisin Custard *(p. 146)*	22%
Peach Kefir Pudding *(p. 151)*	24%
Strawberry Kefir Pudding *(p. 150)*	24%

Sauces & Toppings

Whipped Topping *(p. 159)*	2%
Strawberry Topping *(p. 157)*	5%
Pineapple Topping *(p. 157)*	11%
Fruit Dip *(p. 139)*	22%

MODERATE FAT (31-50%)

Cakes & Frostings

Pineapple Upside-Down Cake (p. 77)	33%
Scripture Fruit Cake (p. 79)	34%
Carrot Cake, unfrosted (p. 67)	35%
Carob Cupcakes, Carob Frosting (p. 68)	38%
Applesauce Cupcake, Cream Cheese Frosting (p. 64)	41%
Applesauce Cake, Cream Cheese Frosting (p. 66)	41%
Date Nut Cake (p. 71)	42%
Chocolate Cupcakes, Chocolate Frosting (p. 68)	43%
Carrot Cake, Cream Cheese Frosting (p. 67)	44%
Carob Cake, unfrosted (p. 70)	46%
Chocolate Cake, unfrosted (p. 70)	47%
Carob Cake, Carob Frosting (p. 70)	50%
No-Bake Honey Cheesecake, reduced fat (p. 76)	50%
Maple Frosting (p. 159)	50%

Candies

Carob Date Fudge (p. 104)	35%
Snowballs (p. 111)	42-43%

Cookies

Carob Brownies (p. 88)	31%
Chocolate No-Bake Cookies (p. 89)	33%
Rice Crispy Oat Cookies, lower fat (p. 110)	33%
Chocolate Brownies (p. 88)	34%
Hobo Fortune Cookies (p. 101)	34%
Emilie's Yummy Oatmeals (p. 97)	36%
Polynesian Squares (p. 109)	36%
Simple Granola Bars (p. 95)	36%
Carob No-Bake Cookies (p. 89)	37%
Tofu Spice Cookies (p. 112)	37%
Frosted Pumpkin Gems (p. 98)	38%
Orange or Lemon Spice Cookies (p. 106)	38%
Persimmon Cookies (p. 108)	39%
Date Almond Granola Bars (p. 95)	40%
Date Walnut Cookies (p. 96)	40%
Kamut-Oatmeal Cookies (p. 102)	40%
Date Sugar Cookies (p. 86)	41%
Emilie's Yummy Oatmeals, coconut (p. 97)	42%
Carob Chip Cookies, oats (p. 90)	42%
Chocolate Chip Cookies, oats (p. 90)	43%
Carob Chip Cookies, no oats (p. 90)	44%
Peanut Butter Sesame Cookies (p. 107)	44%

MODERATE FAT (31-50%), CONT'D
Cookies, Cont'd
Rice Crispy Oat Cookies, higher fat *(p. 110)*	44%
Chocolate Chip Cookies *(p. 90)*	46%
Chocolate Drop Cookies *(p. 92)*	50%

Desserts
Banana Cream Crepes *(p. 137)*	40%
Apple or Peach Crisp *(p. 131)*	41-42%
Strawberry Shortcake, ¼ cup whipped cream *(p. 143)*	47%
Judy's Apple Crisp *(p. 133)*	46-47%

Pies & Pie Crusts
Fresh Apple Pie, single Barley Oat Crust *(p. 120)*	31%
Banana Cream Pie, Meringue, Rice Crust *(p. 122)*	32%
Pumpkin Pie, reduced fat, Barley Oat Crust *(p. 127)*	32%
Pumpkin Pie, reduced fat, Whole Wheat Crust* *(p. 127)*	34%
Lemon Meringue Pie, Rice Crust *(p. 123)*	35%
Lemon Tofu Cheese Pie, Rice Crust *(p. 124)*	35%
Fresh Berry Pie, single Barley Oat Crust *(p. 120)*	36%
Fresh Apple Pie, Whole Wheat Double Crust* *(p. 120)*	38%
Sue's Special Rice Crust *(p. 118)*	39%
Banana Cream Pie, Meringue, Barley Oat Crust *(p. 122)*	39%
Lemon Meringue Pie, Barley Oat Crust *(p. 123)*	39%
Pumpkin Pie, Barley Oat Crust *(p. 127)*	39%
Banana Cream Pie, Meringue, Whole Wheat Crust* *(p. 122)*	42%
Fresh Berry Pie, Whole Wheat Double Crust* *(p. 120)*	42%
Carob Tofu Cheese Pie, Barley Oat Crust *(p. 125)*	43%
Pumpkin Pie, Whole Wheat Crust* *(p. 127)*	43%
Lemon Meringue Pie, Whole Wheat Crust* *(p. 123)*	44%
Carob Tofu Cheese Pie, Whole Wheat Crust* *(p. 125)*	45%
Lemon Tofu Pie, Whole Wheat*, Barley Oat Crust *(p. 123)*	44-46%
Quick Coconut Blender Pie, lowfat milk *(p. 126)*	48%
Heavenly Pecan Pie, Rice Crust *(p. 121)*	49%
Whole Wheat Pie Crust, Pastry Flour *(p. 116-117)*	50%

Puddings & Custards
Almond Millet Custard *(p. 146)*	32%
Vanilla Pudding *(p. 137)*	35%
Berry Non-Dairy Pudding *(p. 159)*	36%
Sweet 'n Spicy Pudding *(p. 152)*	44%

Sauces & Toppings
Joy's 4-in-1 Non-Dairy Sauce *(p. 158)*	36%
Carob Sauce *(p. 156)*	43%
Lemon Sauce *(p. 155)*	47%

*Fat % based on crust made of whole wheat bread flour.

HIGH FAT (51% OR MORE)

Cakes & Frostings
Chocolate Cake, Chocolate Frosting (p. 70)	
German Chocolate Cake (p. 72)	52%
No-Bake Honey Cheesecake (p. 176)	61%
Cream Cheese Frosting (p. 165)	69-75%
Carob Frosting (p. 69)	71%
Chocolate Frosting (p. 69)	75%

Candies
Mother's Little Secret Candies (p. 103)	56-58%
Peanut Clusters (p. 93)	58%
Almond Roca (p. 83)	61-63%

Cookies
Carob Drop Cookies, walnuts (p. 92)	
Candy No-Bake Cookies (p. 87)	52%
Nutty Millet Bars (p. 104)	52%
Cinnamon Crisps (p. 93)	53%
Almond Tea Cakes (p. 84)	56%
Apricot Dream Bars (p. 85)	58%
Coconut Macaroons (p. 94)	62%

Desserts
Apple Walnut Crepes (p. 136)	52%
Honey Vanilla Ice Cream (p. 141)	54%

Pies & Pie Crusts
Heavenly Pecan Pie, Wheat*, Barley Oat Crust (p. 121)	51-53%
Quick Coconut Blender Pie, soy milk (p. 126)	55%
Carob Tofu Cheese Pie, Almond-Coconut Crust (p. 125)	56%
Barley Oat Crust (p. 118)	50%
Graham Cracker Crust (p. 119)	54%
Whole Wheat Pie Crust, bread flour (p. 116-117)	57-58%
Coconut Almond Crust (p. 125)	86%

Puddings
Maple Non-Dairy Pudding (p. 159)	52%
Carob Blanc Mange (p. 145)	59%
Chocolate Blanc Mange (p. 145)	64%

Sauces & Toppings
Chocolate Carob Sauce (p. 156)	51%
Chocolate Sauce, 1 oz. chocolate (p. 156)	57%
Chocolate Sauce, 2 oz. chocolate (p. 156)	60%
Whipped Cream (p. 155)	84%

*Fat % based on crust made of whole wheat bread flour.

About Dairy & Eggs

I recommend nonfat or lowfat milk and yogurt. However, where raw certified milk or pasteurized, non-homogenized yogurt are available (pp. 17-18), I suggest the whole milk product, especially for children. The nutrients of milk and yogurt will be better assimilated and utilized by the body in the presence of the fat. Yogurt should contain live or active cultures.

For nonfat dry milk powder use the non-instant type found in health food stores. Fresh buttermilk is available in supermarkets at fat levels of ½%, 1%, 1½%, and 2% (equivalent of lowfat milk). Powdered buttermilk such as *Darigold* brand is available in health food stores. Some supermarkets carry a powdered buttermilk culture under the brand name called *Seco*.

Excellent non-dairy replacements for milk in dessert recipes include *Rice Dream Non Dairy Beverage* (made from brown rice, safflower oil, and salt), and soy milk (especially *Better Than Milk*, a tofu non-dairy beverage manufactured by Sovex Natural Foods, Inc.) *Better Than Milk Tofu Beverage* is my first choice as a non-dairy alternative. These may be purchased at most health food stores. For more information on dairy and non-dairy alternatives see **Breakfasts**, *Milk Alternatives*, pp. 21-29. Fruit juices, such as apple and pineapple juice, work with varying degrees of success in baked goods in place of milk.

Eggs act as a binder of ingredients in baking, add high quality protein and fat, and small amounts of a variety of vitamins and minerals. Two egg whites may be substituted for each egg used in any recipe. *Egg Beaters*, which are essentially egg whites, may also be used in proportion listed on the box. Totally eggless alternatives and other kinds of eggs include flaxseed binder, arrowroot binder, tofu, *Ener-G Egg Replacer*, quail eggs, and duck eggs (see **Breakfasts**, p. 269 for information on these alternatives). In baked goods *Flaxseed Binder*, **Breakfasts**, p. 269, is an especially nutritious and successful egg replacement. See also *Fat and Egg Substitute Products*, p. 33.

About Fruits & Juices

Fruits, Canned

I do not recommend the liberal use of canned fruits, because they have undergone considerable heat processing. Consequently, the nutritional value is reduced. Whenever canned fruits are called for, purchase fruits not sweetened with refined sugars. The fruit juice alone in canned fruits is adequate sweetening without additional sugar. Several brands of fruits packed in their own juice or a combination of concentrated fruit juices are readily available in supermarkets. These are usually labeled "In Its Own Juice" (or Juices). Make certain that they are not also "lightly sweetened." That means corn syrup and/or sugar has probably been added. You probably won't find this on the front of the can. Check the small print ingredients label. Unsweetened pineapple and apple-sauce are clearly labeled on the front of the can or jar, but it is easy to pick up the sweetened variety if you don't read the label as these are stocked side-by-side on supermarket shelves.

For home canning of fruits, a light syrup using honey in place of sugar works well. Use half the amount of honey as sugar, following the same canning procedure recommended in a home canning guide. Use a mild flavored honey.

Fruits, Dried

Drying fruits retains the nutrients in the fresh fruit. Minerals and fruit sugars are concentrated. Most dried fruits in supermarkets are treated with sulfur dioxide to retain the bright original color. If you compare sulfured apricots with unsulfured apricots, for example, you will notice how dark the latter are. The problem with sulfur is that it puts stress on the kidneys. It also affects the pH balance of the fruits, shifting the effect of the fruit on the blood pH from alkaline to acidic. Since our typical diet errs on the side of too many acid producing foods, it is wise to select unsulfured dried fruits. When dried fruit is softened in water and then added to a dessert, the color contrast between sulfured and unsulfured is not so noticeable.

Other dried fruit additives include sorbic acid and corn syrup (some health food store offerings have honey added). Date dices are often coated in sugar. Dried fruits need neither preservatives nor sugars of any kind. Anything that is added to dried fruits must be listed on the label. It is not difficult to buy dark raisins (as Thompson seedless) in supermarkets that are sun dried without any sulfur dioxide or other additions, but for most other dried fruits you will need to rely on a health food store, mail order source, or food co-op. Most health food stores carry date dices or nuggets coated in oat flour instead of sugar.

Fruits, Frozen

Purchase unsweetened frozen fruits. These are readily available, but read package labels carefully. If you want unsweetened frozen strawberries, they will probably be whole berries. I have yet to see frozen sliced strawberries that are not sweetened. Whole frozen strawberries are easily sliced when slightly thawed.

More nutrients are retained in frozen than in canned fruits, while dried fruits retain the most. Whenever a recipe gives the choice of fresh or frozen fruit, choose the fresh. The flavor will be better and the cost usually less.

Fruit Juices

You will find a broad range of both canned and frozen unsweetened juices in both supermarkets and health food stores. Read labels carefully to make sure no sweeteners have been added. Beware of a label that says "all natural." Refined sugars qualify as "natural ingredients."

Fruit Spreads

All fruit or 100% fruit spreads or jams are now available in supermarkets as well as health food stores. Those in supermarkets are generally lower in price. These are quite tasty and the added sugar is hardly missed. Health food stores also carry honey-sweetened jam.

About Carob, Chocolate & Cocoa

The streets of my neighborhood are lined with carob trees. The enterprising founder of our city planted acres of them. Unfortunately there was little commercial demand for carob. Fortunately the carob tree in front of our house is male. Thus, our sidewalk doesn't get littered with the hard, dried, dark brown pods. I've saved an article on file with instructions for processing carob from the pods to make them edible in case of famine. I assure you that otherwise it would not be worth the effort!

The carob tree is also known as a locust tree. Because the John the Baptist ate locusts and wild honey, carob is often called St. John's bread. Nutritious it is! Carob is a legume and thus its protein content complements the protein of whole grain flours. It is a good source of pectin which is a valuable dietary fiber, and calcium. Carob contains 92 mg. calcium per 3 tablespoons, 4 times that of an equivalent amount of chocolate. In addition, carob contains a mere 0.4 grams fat per 3 tablespoons as compared to the equivalent 1 oz. chocolate with 14.6 grams fat.

If you are a chocolate connoisseur, the flavor of carob may not satisfy you. But do give it a try. Recipes in **Desserts** give you both alternatives. The equivalent of carob to chocolate is:

3 Tbsps. carob + 2 Tbsp. water = 1 oz. unsweetened chocolate

The hot water blended with the carob is equivalent to a melted chocolate square, or the dry powder can be added to the dry ingredients and the water added to the liquids. To substitute carob powder for cocoa use the same amount. Since carob is not as bitter as chocolate or cocoa a recipe with carob may require a little less sweetening. For best flavor, purchase carob powder that is roasted. It is available both in supermarkets and health food stores.

Is chocolate really bad for you? Yes, if you are a chocolate lover who "eats a chocolate bar a day, it might not keep the doctor away." Besides being a poor source of calcium, the oxalic acid content of chocolate can interfere with the absorption of calcium. It can also prevent absorption of some B-vitamins, most notably the anti-stress B-vitamins. Chocolate can also decrease the effectiveness of some medications and aggravate allergy symptoms. Quite high in fat, chocolate also contains a good portion of caffeine. But help is on the way! A new product, *WonderSlim Low-Fat Cocoa Powder*, is fat free and 99.7% caffeine free (see p. 18). It works and tastes just like regular cocoa powder in recipes. Look for it in health food stores, and eventually in some supermarkets. Unless you are allergic to chocolate itself, or unless it aggravates other allergy symptoms or interferes with some medication, an occasional dessert with chocolate will probably do little harm. Enjoy it!

Carob Chips

Carob chips may be purchased sweetened or unsweetened. I recommend the unsweetened. *Sunspire*, available at health food stores, is an excellent choice containing carob powder, whey powder, nonfat milk powder, fractionated palm kernel oil, and lecithin. Fractionated palm oil is not hydrogenated. Fractionated processing produces a purer oil. Forty five percent of the calories in carob chips come from fat.

About Coconut

Dried coconut is another food that needs no added sugar to enhance flavor. Yet, unsweetened coconut is practically nonexistent in supermarkets. Most health food stores carry unsweetened coconut at very reasonable prices, usually in 1 lb. bags. Different particle sizes of coconut go under different names such as macaroon or fine shred, thread or medium shred, chip or coarse shred. Macaroon or fine shred coconut designates tiny pieces almost like a meal. Thread or medium shred coconut looks like grated cheese. Chip or coarse shred coconut is cut in short fat pieces that look like wood shavings.

Because coconut is high in fat, it should be stored carefully. As long as it is unopened, dried coconut will keep at room temperature up to 6 months. After opening, it keeps 3-4 weeks in the refrigerator or up to 6 months in the freezer.

About Nuts & Seeds

Do not avoid nuts and seeds because they are high in fat. The latest research indicates that people who eat several handfuls of nuts a week have less heart disease than those who don't eat nuts. Why is this? First of all, the fat is primarily unsaturated and is dispursed throughout an unrefined whole food rather than concentrated as an oil. Secondly, nuts contain vitamin E and a wide range of nutrients plus fiber. These all work together synergistically (see **Breakfasts**, p. 55) to provide excellent nutritional value. I often reduce the nuts from original recipes to half the amount to reduce the fat content and cost, but seldom omit them entirely.

Purchase unsalted and unroasted nuts and seeds. These may be found in supermarkets in small quantities for a high price. More economical sizes and prices are available in health food stores, through mail order or food co-ops. Roasted nuts used in **Desserts** are peanuts, and occasionally almonds. Both are best home-toasted (see pp. 73, 93, 103). Store all shelled nuts and seeds in airtight bags or containers in the refrigerator or freezer. Most keep 6-9 months in refrigerator or 9-12 months in the freezer. There may be some loss of flavor and crunch in freezer storage, but you probably won't notice the difference. It is best not to keep any shelled nuts or seeds at room temperature over a few days.

Peanut Butter

Most peanut butter in supermarkets contains partially hydrogenated fat and refined sugar. *Laura Scudders* or other selected brands in supermarkets contain only peanuts and salt. Peanut butter made from peanuts alone, with or without salt, is available in most health food stores. When first opened, peanut butter without hydrogenated fat will have a layer of oil that has separated and risen to the top of the jar. Scoop the contents of the jar into a mixing bowl, blend it well, and return it to the jar. Usually it will not separate again. Keep refrigerated after opening, up to 3-4 months for commerical peanut butter, or 10 days if homemade.

About Spices & Flavorings

More spice is needed to bring out the flavor when baking with whole grain flours. When changing a white flour recipe to whole grain flour, I double the amount of spice (but not the flavoring), give it the taste test and then adjust accordingly. I use the supermarket spices and flavorings. Most extracts are sugar-free, but read labels if concerned about this. A few do contain it. Pure vanilla contains sugar. *Cook's Choice*, a brand of vanilla in health food stores is sugar-free.

About Leavenings & Thickenings

Leavening is the ingredient that causes the baked product to rise during baking. In quick breads (breads made without yeast) baking powder and baking soda are used. Beaten egg whites also help to leaven baked foods.

Baking powder and soda can alter the pH balance of the batter so that some of the B-vitamins are destroyed if too much is used. This can be minimized by keeping the amount of leavening to 1 teaspoon per 1 cup flour. For example, if a recipe calls for 2½ cups flour, use 2½ teaspoons leavening. With this limitation I have found that a little baking soda used in combination with baking powder produces better rising results--usually about ½ teapsoon baking soda. Soda is much higher in sodium content, however, than baking powder. If you are on a salt-restricted diet, you can use 1½ teaspoons low sodium baking powder in place of ½ teaspoon baking soda.

Leavenings should be fresh and active to give satisfactory results. For a fuller explanation of leavenings, testing freshness, and homemade baking powder recipes, see *Breakfasts*, pp. 278-280.

Low Sodium Baking Powder

Low sodium baking powder, available at most health food stores, is my first choice for quality. It contains no aluminum or corn, and just 1.5 mg. sodium per teaspoon as compared to over 300 mg. sodium per teaspoon of regular double acting baking powder. Nutrient data for sodium in all our recipes is based on using low sodium baking powder.

Label instructions for low sodium baking powder suggest using 1½ teaspoons to replace 1 teaspoon regular baking powder. However, I just use 1 teaspoon low sodium baking powder to replace 1 teaspoon regular baking powder.

Rumford Baking Powder

Rumford Baking Powder, though containing corn and not low sodium, is aluminum-free as a second better alternative to regular baking powder. It is available in most health food stores and in some supermarkets.

Arrowroot Powder and Cornstarch

Arrowroot is a starch that comes from the tubers of several tropical plants. It contains trace minerals and is therefore of better nutritional quality than cornstarch. Arrowroot requires a lower cooking temperature than cornstarch, and a shorter cooking time. Thus, more care is necessary to achieve success when using it. It does not hold up as well when reheated.

Arrowroot is more expensive than cornstarch. Since it is used in such small amounts, however, the added expense is minor. One pound packages available at health food stores are more economical than the small jars available at supermarkets.

Cornstarch comes from the endosperm of the corn kernel. It can be used interchangeably with arrowroot powder. Arrowroot or cornstarch should always be blended into room temperature or cool liquid before heating to prevent lumps. While heating over moderately low heat, whisk gently but constantly. When mixture comes to a boil (arrowroot should be brought barely to a boil), do not boil over 1 minute. When eggs are to be added, some of the hot mixture is stirred into the eggs and then the egg mixture stirred back into the pot. It is then cooked at boiling temperature 1 minute longer. Acid ingredients such as lemon juice hinder the thickening process and thus should not be added during cooking but after mixture is thickened and removed from the heat. Stir acid ingredients in gently.

A double boiler is ideal for cooking puddings and pie fillings thickened with arrowroot or cornstarch, especially if you have poor quality saucepans (see p. 47). If you have problems with thickening puddings with the few guidelines here, you might want to read more thorough how-to instructions with cornstarch and arrowroot in *Joy of Cooking* (look up cornstarch and arrowroot in the index).

Unflavored Gelatine

Gelatine is a good source of incomplete protein. One envelope (¼ oz.) adequately thickens 2 cups of liquid. For making jello cubes use 1 envelope to 1½ cups liquid. Too much gelatine will produce a rubbery texture. It may be dissolved directly in boiling liquid, but I prefer softening it in cold or room temperature liquid for about 5 minutes before dissolving over heat. This method guarantees complete dissolving and effective gelling.

A small box of *Knox* gelatine contains 4 envelopes; a large box contains 32 envelopes. Both are available in supermarkets. If you purchase gelatine in bulk, use 2 teaspoons for a recipe calling for 1 envelope. If a recipe calls for 1½ envelopes, use 1 tablespoon (2 tsps.= 1 envelope; 1 tsp.= ½ envelope).

Preparation & Baking How To's

BAKEWARE & UTENSILS

Purchasing Quality

Aluminum has been linked to Alzheimer's disease in recent years. Definitive studies have not settled this issue. Consequently many cooks are questioning the use of aluminum cookware. I recommend minimizing its use in food preparation in the following ways:

~ Avoid cooking acid-based foods (i.e. tomatoes) in aluminum cookware. The acid reacts with the metal.

~ Wrap foods to be frozen in saran wrap before wrapping in aluminum foil.

~ Use a baking powder that does not contain aluminum (p.44).

~ Purchase most of your cookware made with alternative metals and pyrex glass (see below).

~ Don't worry about the occasional use of bake pans that aren't readily available in anything but aluminum (i.e. angel tube cake pans).

Purchase as much bakeware as possible in either stainless steel or pyrex glass. Pyrex glass loaf pans, pie plates, and square or rectangle cake pans are readily available. Pyrex glass pans are very durable (I haven't broken one yet) and are easy to clean. More stainless steel bakeware than ever is available, even cookie sheets and muffin or cupcake pans. The double thick insulated cookie sheets especially protect cookies from burning and uneven baking, but I have only found them in aluminum.

APPLIANCES

Blender

For desserts I use the blender for crepe batter, blending cream cheese, sour cream, and yogurts. It is also handy for nut grinding and making graham cracker crumbs, although I prefer a hand method for making cracker crumbs and a chef's knife for chopping nuts. A blender has so many other effective and timesaving uses, not to speak of *Whole Grain Blender Magic* and wonderful *Meals-in-a-glass* blender shakes (**Breakfasts**). A good blender that will crush ice cubes, in the $40 range, is a blessing to have in every kitchen.

Electric mixer

An upright table model is much faster than a hand-held one, and more effective. I use the electric mixer for desserts to beat egg whites, whip cream and topping, and mix frostings and angel food cake.

SAUCEPANS

Basic set stainless steel waterless cookware

High quality lifetime waterless cookware pots and pans are admittedly expensive, but well worth the investment. High quality cookware is constructed of inner layers of aluminum with outer layers of surgical stainless steel for optimum heat distribution. Layers distributed throughout the sides and bottom of the pans heat more evenly than layers on the bottom only. *Saladmaster* cookware, marketed through home parties, is an example of this construction (see p. 17). Other companies also market waterless cookware.

Double boiler

A double boiler combines a top pan for cooking that fits inside a bottom pan that holds water. This keeps the pan surface in which the food is cooked away from direct heat to prevent burning, boiling over, and overcooking. It is especially useful for cooking puddings containing milk, eggs, and cornstarch or arrowroot as a thickener. While not an absolute essential, it is a useful addition to a saucepan set.

BAKING PANS

9" x 13" bake pan (one with a lid is handy for transporting)

8" or 9" square bake pan

3 - 9" layer cake pans: for *German Chocolate Cake* (p. 72)

bundt pan: scalloped pan for unfrosted cakes *(see Serving Desserts, p. 57)*

angel tube cake pan: for *Angel Food, Orange Chiffon Cakes* (pp. 68, 75)

12 cup cupcake (muffin) pan: with wells 3" diameter x 1¼" deep

2 cookie sheets: for rotating through oven; insulated type is
    excellent for quality cookies, although made of aluminum

9" or 9½" pie plate: I prefer 9½" size (available in pyrex glass)

2 - 8½" x 4½" medium loaf pans:
  1 for *Nut Bread*, 2 for *Scripture Fruit Cake* (pp. 140, 79)
  or **3 - 6 mini-loaf pans:** 3 are equivalent to 1 medium
  loaf pan; these are 5¾" x 3" x 21/8"

6" - 8" crepe pan: for *Dessert Crepes* (p. 135)

UTENSILS

mixing bowl set of 3: small/med/lg (stainless or pyrex glass).

wire whisks: At least one! 1 large, 1 medium, 1 mini-size are
better; for blending liquid ingredients, thin batters, stirring
puddings.

rubber spatulas: The curved *Rubbermaid Spoonula* is especially
effective and serves also as a spoon and a scoop, reducing
number of utensils often needed for mixing and filling bake
pans. Look for these in kitchen specialty shops and restaurant
supply outlets.

large mixing spoon: May be wooden, but large stainless steel
serving spoons from a flatware set work better.

measuring spoons: I recommend *EZ Measure* by *Mirro* in 2 adjust-
able sizes: 1 tsp-1 Tbsp. and 1/8 tsp.-1 tsp. A lever adjusts the
measure. The smaller spoon fits into narrow-mouthed spice jars.

nest of measuring cups: For dry ingredients. *Tupperware*
includes 2/3 cup and ¾ cup measures; 1/8 cup measure
(2 Tbsps.) is very handy and can usually be purchased as
a single item; coffee scoops are usually this size.

1 and 2 cup measuring cups for liquids: Pyrex glass or see-through
plastic, clearly marked; when marks wear away through use,
remark with an indelible felt tip marker.

egg separator: Separates yolks from whites; available through
Tupperware, kitchen specialty shops.

oven thermometer: For accurate baking temperature; oven dials
are often not accurate; purchase in a supermarket.

all-purpose scoop dispenser: For cookie dough; looks like a
mini-ice cream scoop; I use a 1" scoop (holds 1 Tbsp. dough);
available in specialty housewares shops; if you want to make
your cookies larger than this standard size, purchase a larger
scoop (p. 55).

metal spatula: These are getting harder to find, 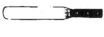 but are especially helpful for spreading frosting on cakes and leveling dry ingredients when measuring; check in housewares shops.

rolling pin: For pie crusts.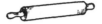

pie server: Wedge shaped for pies, layer cakes.

pastry sheet: Such as tupperware, for rolling out pie crusts; not essential if crusts are rolled between two pieces wax paper, but still nice to lay underneath.

chef's knife: Speeds chopping of nuts, dried fruit, fresh fruit and vegetables; purchase at a restaurant supply store for sturdy quality, reasonable price, and helpful service; 8" or 10" long.

kitchen timer: Save many a burned cookie! Buy one that won't break in less than a year, such as a digital timer.

lemon/orange zester: Much easier than using a grater; check in housewares shop.

pastry blender: Cut butter into flour for pie crusts (although 2 table knives will do).

strainers: 1 large, 1 small; these make great simple sifters (p. 51).

kitchen shears: Cut up dates, figs, trim pie crusts.

candy thermometer: For *Almond Roca* (p. 83).

MEASURING & MIXING INGREDIENTS

Measuring

For good results in baking, measurements need to be accurate. Standard measuring spoons and cups are essential. Dry ingredients should be evenly leveled off at the rim of the measure. Thus a measuring cup used for liquids where the necessary measurement line is not at the rim is not appropriate for dry ingredients. A nest of dry measuring cups serves the purpose. A 2/3 cup and ¾ cup measure are good additions (available through *Tupperware*). In addition, get a 1/8 cup measure which is seldom in a set, but very handy. These are readily available in supermarkets. Coffee scoops also usually make good 1/8 cup measures (check out the volume to be sure--1/8 cup = 2 Tbsps.).

Traditional cookbooks instruct cooks to measure the flour after sifting because it measures differently after sifting than before. I don't sift whole grain flour. In fact, I do not even own a sifter. Therefore, all our recipes (except *Angel Food Cake*) assume measurement of unsifted flour. To measure whole grain flour dip the measuring cup into the flour and scoop it lightly into the cup. Without packing it down, level it off with your finger, a metal spatula, or straight edge of a table knife.

To measure dry ingredients such as baking powder, baking soda, salt, and spices, I recommend dipping the measuring spoon into the container and leveling it off with either a finger or the edge of the container. This is much easier than pouring from the container into the measuring spoon. The 1/8 tsp.-1 tsp. *EZ Measure* by *Mirro* (see measuring spoons, p. 48) is ideal for this. If your measuring spoon does not fit into a narrow-mouthed spice jar, transfer the spice to another container, or dip in a smaller measure twice (e.g. dip the ½ tsp. measure into the jar two times to make 1 tsp.).

To measure honey, when using oil measure the oil in the same cup first; then the honey will slide right out of the measuring cup. If using melted butter, pour some into the measuring cup to "grease it", pour out, and measure honey to slide right out. If using neither oil or melted butter, spray the measuring cup with non-stick spray first (not as effective, but it helps). If the honey does not pour easily from the container to the measuring cup (a problem especially in cold weather), warm the honey container, if it is not metal, in the microwave about 20 - 40 seconds.

You can save yourself a lot of time by memorizing the measurement equivalents below. By doing so you can choose the measure that is most efficient that is equivalent to what is listed in a recipe. You will also then know how to conveniently measure a divided or multiplied recipe. Below is a brief list. For a more complete list of equivalents, see **Main Dishes**, pp. 56-67.

1½ tsps. = ½ Tbsp.	3/8 cup = 6 Tbsps.
3 tsps. = 1 Tbsp.	½ cup = 8 Tbsps.
2 Tbsps. = 1/8 cup	5/8 cup = 10 Tbsps.
¼ cup = 4 Tbsps	16 Tbsps. = 1 cup
1/3 cup = 5 1/3 Tbsps.	

Here is an example of how you can apply your knowledge of equivalents to our recipes. When **Desserts** recipes require 1 tablespoon baking powder, 3 teaspoons baking powder is listed to prevent the easy mistake of reading 1 tablespoon as 1 teaspoon. Yet, it will be quicker to measure the 3 teaspoons with the 1 tablespoon measure.

Memorize the equivalent of liquid measure to weight listed below. This will not usually apply to dry ingredients or highly viscous liquids such as honey, but is very helpful in purchasing and measuring canned liquids such as fruit juices or evaporated milk, and most 16 oz. cans of fruit. For example, a 6 oz. can of pineapple juice is ¾ cup, and a 12 oz. can evaporated milk is 1½ cups.

16 oz. can = 2 cups canned fruit with juice
1½ cups liquid = 12 fluid ounces
1 cup liquid = 8 fluid ounces
¾ cup liquid = 6 fluid ounces

One rather surprising measurement equivalent helpful to know, especially for shopping is that 1 lb. (16 oz.) honey measures only 11/3 cups, not 2 cups as most other liquids. So if you are buying honey for a recipe that calls for 2 cups, 1 lb. or 16 oz. won't do. It still amazes me how quickly 3 lbs. of honey disappear!

A few other equivalents you will find useful to memorize are:
1 stick butter = ½ cup; 1 lb. butter (4 sticks) = 2 cups
8 oz. can pineapple with juice = 1 cup
20 oz. can pineapple with juice = 2½ cups
6 oz. chocolate or carob chips = 1 cup; 12 oz. = 2 cups

Mixing Dry Ingredients

There are several dry ingredients used in baking that may have lumps in them that need to be sieved before adding them to the recipe for smooth and even mixing. This is especially true of ingredients without any additive to keep them free flowing (such as sea salt). For these, I measure the ingredient, place it in a strainer over the mixing bowl and stir it through the strainer with a spoon. This quickly breaks up any lumps. Once all the lumps are gone, if any of the ingredient remains in the strainer, I just turn the strainer over and dump the rest into the bowl--no need to keep stirring until the last bits of ingredient fall through the strainer if all the lumps are already dispersed! For this process I use either a large or small strainer. Below is a list of ingredients that might have lumps where a strainer comes in handy.

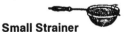

Small Strainer
baking soda
baking powder
salt (a quality sea salt
    such as *RealSalt*
    clumps easily)

Large Strainer
crystalline fructose
Sucanat (lumpy on occasion)
cocoa or carob powder
nonfat non-instant dry milk powder
arrowroot powder or cornstarch

I also use a large strainer to lighten flour for *Angel Food Cake*. Since the bran will not go through the strainer, however, after stirring all the flour through the strainer, I turn the strainer over and dump in the bran with its valuable nutrients and fiber.

If flour has been kept refrigerated, bring it to room temperature for baking cakes, cupcakes, or quick loaf breads. For cookies and pie crusts it will work well if still at refrigerator-cold temperature.

Stir dry ingredients in mixing bowl together thoroughly to blend evenly before combining with liquid ingredients.

Mixing Liquid Ingredients

To keep mixing bowls from clattering and slipping while mixing ingredients by hand, put a folded towel on the counter top underneath them. You will be surprised how helpful this simple step is!

Except for most cakes, I mix by hand. With the help of a wire whisk, hand mixing is just as fast, and you are less likely to overmix. A key to easy hand mixing is to switch utensils to suit the stiffness of batter or dough. The wire whisk works wonderfully to quickly blend liquid ingredients. One exception is when a granular sweetener, such as *Sucanat*, is added to liquid; sometimes I switch to a spoon to mix it in because the batter is momentarily too stiff for the whisk and just clogs it up. I would rather use an extra utensil and save hassle while I am mixing.

Proper preparation of ingredients will facilitate quick and thorough blending. For example, you will often read in cookbooks the term, *cream the butter and sugar.* Our grandmothers knew what this meant, but few cooks today know what it means. It means to beat the sugar and butter or shortening together until thoroughly blended and creamy. In **Desserts** I use the word "whisk" in place of "cream," a reminder to use a whisk. It also helps to have the butter very soft before adding the sugar. If it is hard, I put it in the microwave on about #3 power until it is very soft but not melted, then whisk it in the mixing bowl vigorously before blending in the sweetener. If the mixture is too stiff for a whisk, I switch to a spoon.

The remaining liquid ingredients are easily whisked into the "creamed" butter and sugar. Milk or juice should not be blended in too vigorously as curdling of the ingredients sometimes then occurs. In cakes, milk is usually added alternately to remaining liquid ingredients with the dry ingredients.

52

Blending Liquid & Dry Ingredients

In making cookies dry ingredients are usually added to the liquid ingredients. For pie crusts liquid ingredients are added to the dry ingredients. For cakes dry ingredients are added alternately with the milk (if any) to liquid ingredients. Overmixing dry ingredients with liquid ingredients is a frequent mistake. Stir or fold liquid ingredients into dry ingredients just until mixed. Overmixing develops the gluten in the flour and produces a heavier texture, especially in cookies and pie crusts. If the batter or dough is quite stiff, a mixing spoon works best. If the mixture is fairly soft and smooth, the curved *Rubbermaid Spoonula* (see p. 48) works great for a combination of folding and stirring. Cake batters can be beaten a little more vigorously since there is less flour and you want it dispersed smoothly and evenly throughtout the liquid ingredients.

For pie crusts, use a pastry blender or 2 table knives to work in the fat, and a fork to stir in the ice water. The key to all blending of ingredients is to use the most effective and efficient tool for the job.

Separating, Beating, Folding in Egg Whites

Incredibly, some cooks have never learned to separate an egg! Eggs are usually separated in order to beat up the whites to make a lighter baked product. The rule is to never allow any egg yolk to get into the egg white. I seldom use the word "never," but it does apply for successful beating of egg whites. They will not beat stiff if any yolk is present. The first step of prevention is to separate eggs while they are refrigerator-cold. Room temperature egg yolks break too easily.

The old-fashioned method is to break the egg shell in half on the side of the bowl, then pour the egg yolk from one half the egg shell to the other, allowing the white to escape to a container underneath. A surer and easier method is to do it with an egg separator (see p. 48). Set the egg separator over a small container with an edge that the separator can rest on easily and break the egg into it. Pick the separator up and tip from side to side to allow the white to run out the open sides. Place the yolk in a separate container. Pour the white you just separated into the mixing bowl before you separate another egg. Thus, if yolk lands in the next white, you haven't ruined all you have already separated. If I ruin a white, I usually just add it into the recipe with the yolks. When unbeaten egg whites are called for, a little yolk present in them is not important.

While eggs are best separated at refrigerator-cold temperature, egg whites beat up stiff in higher volumn if first brought to room temperature. Allow time after separation for the whites to come to room temperature before beating them up. This will be especially helpful when making *Angel Food* or *Orange Chiffon Cake* (p. 68, 75). Egg whites are best beaten at high speed in an electric mixer (not a blender). Any sweetening to be added is usually gradually added after whites are beaten to the foamy stage. Cream of tartar is often added to produce firmer, more stable, stiffly beaten egg whites.

Egg whites are properly beaten stiff when they will hold firm, upright peaks. Overbeaten egg whites will not hold together well and will seem dry. You'll know if you've overbeaten them. Fold beaten egg whites gently into batter with a rubber spatula.

Cooking with Eggs

Whole eggs or egg yolks are often used in puddings. To prevent overcooking of eggs, the first stage of cooking the pudding is done without them. A small amount of hot pudding is then gradually whisked into the slightly beaten eggs. This mixture is then gradually whisked back into the hot pudding remaining in the saucepan for another minute of cooking. This method prevents the egg from turning into cooked egg "pieces" in the pudding. When cooking puddings, a double boiler is very helpful (see p. 47).

BAKING TIPS

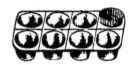

Preparing Bake Pans

When dry and liquid ingredients have been combined, the leavening is activated and the batter should go into the oven as soon as possible for best results (with exception of cookies and pie crusts). Thus, have the bake pans prepared in advance--greased, sprayed, lined with wax paper or with paper bake cups. This is essential primarily for cakes, cupcakes, quick loaf breads, and muffins that contain baking powder.

The quickest greasing method for bake pans is to use a non-stick spray. I recommend using an olive oil-based non-stick spray such as *Pam*, available in many supermarkets and most health food stores. Pans may also be greased with a blend of about 1 part liquid lecithin and 2 parts oil. While butter alone prevents sticking, oil will not. Lecithin is one of the ingredients used in non-stick spray. It is a highly nutritions part of the soybean. Liquid lecithin may be purchased at health food stores. It may seem expensive, but a little goes a long way and it will keep almost indefinitely in the cupboard. Pour a small amount in the bake pan, add a little oil and spread together evenly around the pan with a piece of wax paper.

For cakes that are to be removed from the pans (such as layered *German Chocolate Cake*, or *Scripture Cake*, lining the bottom of the pans with wax paper is an added guarantee that the cake will come out easily. Tear off a piece of wax paper a little larger than the pan bottom. Set the pan on top of it on the counter and draw a line around the edge of the pan on the wax paper either with a pencil or the point of the kitchen shears. With the shears, cut the pan shape just inside the marking; it should fit just about right. For insurance, I lightly spray the pan under and on top of the wax paper.

If you use paper bake cups for cupcakes, lightly spray the insides with non-stick spray anyway. This will facilitate pealing the paper off the baked cupcake.

Filling Pans

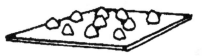

When baking with whole grain flours, pans are usually filled with more batter since whole grain baked goods do not rise high. All the recipes in **Desserts** have been tested with the size pans listed in the recipes. If you bake cupcakes using paper bake cups you will probably need more than one 12-cup muffin pan for a cupcake recipe, since paper bake cups cannot be filled as full as unlined muffin cups.

When dropping cookie dough on cookie sheets, leaving about 2" between cookies is a good habit whether the cookies spread or not. I use a 1" all-purpose scoop dispenser (p. 48) for drop cookies and as a shaper for cookie dough that would otherwise be rolled in the palms of the hands. A real boon to cookie making, the scoop dispenser is much faster, produces cookies of uniform size, and eliminates the need for chilling dough for easier handling. As a rolled cookie shaper, it is quicker than rolling the dough in the palms of the hands. Use two cookie sheets to rotate through the oven--when one pan comes out have another ready to go in.

Preheating Oven

The oven should be preheated to full temperature before baking. Unless some steps are to be done at an earlier time, the best time to turn the oven on is just before you assemble the ingredients. Know how long your own oven requires to preheat.

If you use a glass pan for a recipe calling for 350° or higher, lower the temperature by 25° since glass absorbs more heat than metal. Likewise, if you substitute honey in a recipe calling for sugar, lower the heat by 25°. In either case, do not lower the oven temperature below 325°. When making these adjustments, be aware that the time needed to bake may change by a few minutes. Make adjustment notes on your recipes.

Be sure to get an oven thermometer to hang or set permanently in your oven where you can easily read it without having to move it to put pans in. Many ovens, especially the older gas ovens, easily vary in actual temperature from the reading on the dial by 25° or so. The consequences can be frustrating! Oven thermometers, readily available in supermarkets, are inexpensive insurance.

Baking

Most baked goods will bake more evenly if baked in the center of the oven with some room all around the pan for air circulation. Raise or lower one of the oven racks to the center of the oven. Bake only one sheet of cookies at a time for best results since cookie sheets take up a lot of shelf space. Two pie pans, or 3 round layer cake pans, or 4-6 medium loaf or 6-8 mini-loaf pans will fit well on one shelf in a 30" oven with sufficient circulating room around each pan.

If you want to use both oven racks for baking, expect what is on the top rack to get browned on top before it is done in the center. Expect what is on the bottom shelf to get sufficiently browned on the bottom before it is done in the center. One way to avoid over-browning on top or bottom is to rotate items on top and bottom racks--about 2/3 the way through baking time for cakes, or halfway through baking time for cookies or pies.

Even though recipes suggest the length of baking time, you will get better results by using an additional test for doneness. For cakes or quick breads, use a clean knife or toothpick inserted in the center. If it comes out clean, the cake or bread is done. An additional test for cakes is whether cake has pulled away from sides of the pan. If a cake browns on the surface more than you want it before it is done in the center, make a note on your recipe to lower the temperature a bit the next time you bake it (see last paragraph, p. 55).

The best test for doneness of cookies is the color. They should be a delicately light golden brown unless you like them more done. The firmness of the cookie is not always a good guide. Some recipes are quite soft while hot, but firm up as they cool. When baking cookies I always set the timer for the shorter length of time suggested in the recipe to check doneness at that point.

The color of cookie sheets affects how quickly cookies turn dark. If the metal is light they will brown more slowly; if the sheet is darkened, more quickly. I find that I need to bake the same recipe of cookies 1 or 2 minutes less on my older cookie sheets (darker with age) than the newer ones.

When baking pies, if the edge of the crust begins to get too brown before the filling is done, lightly cover the edges with foil.

Cooling

Some cookies will fall apart if immediately removed from the cookie sheet. They need to firm up with cooling. Others are best removed immediately. Instructions for when to remove cookies in *Desserts* are given with each recipe. Always cool cookies without stacking them. Cool them on a wood counter top, wooden cutting board, cooling rack, or cut a brown paper sack to place them on. Let cookies cool entirely before stacking them on top of one another.

Cool quick loaf breads in the pans 10 minutes, then turn them out of the pans onto their sides on a cooling rack, wood counter top, or wooden cutting board. Let them cool completely before slicing.

Let cakes cool in the pan about 10 minutes. Then cool cake layers on cooling racks, right side up, leaving the wax paper on the bottom until ready to assemble. Otherwise, the cake will probably stick to the surface it is cooled on. For bundt cakes, remove directly from the pan to the serving plate. For angel food cake follow the cooling instructions for the recipe. All cakes and cookies should be entirely cooled before frosting.

Puddings continue to thicken upon cooling, so don't worry if they haven't thickened to the consistency you desire within the length of cooking time suggested. This is especially important because overcooked cornstarch or arrowroot will not produce the desired texture. If you cook tapioca to the point you desire, it will probably thicken beyond what you want when it is cold.

Serving Desserts

Cutting cakes: Since we often serve cake unfrosted, I enjoy using a bundt pan instead of a 9" x 13" pan. When cut into servings the bundt cake has a gourmet look, especially if topped with whipped cream, ice cream, berries, or a fruit sauce. Bundt cakes are simple to cut into even sized pieces. For 24 servings, cut each wide scallop into two pieces, and make each narrow scallop one piece.

A 9" x 13" cake easily serves 18. Cut the cake 3 x 6, cutting it in thirds lengthwise. To cut width of cake evenly into sixths, cut width in half first; then cut each half evenly 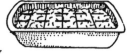 into thirds. For smaller servings cut cake 4 x 6 (24 servings per 9" x 13" pan). For an 8" or 9" square cake, cut it 4 x 4, 3 x 4, or 3 x 3 depending on whether you want very small, medium, or very large pieces. Angel food, chiffon, and layer cakes serve at least 12.

Serving Cookies   The flavor of many cookies in this book is improved by allowing them to get quite cold in the refrigerator or freezer. Remove cookies from the freezer just a few minutes before serving. The number of cookies a **Desserts** recipe makes is based on measuring the dough with a 1" scoop dispenser (p. 48), or about 1 tablespoon dough per cookie. The cookies will be small except for some that spread out a lot. I recommend serving a greater number of smaller cookies than fewer large ones. Children, especially, will think they are getting more that way--and some adults, too!

Storing Desserts

The more sugar a recipe contains, the longer the shelf life since sugar acts as a preservative. One of the reasons that sugar is found in so many packaged foods is to increase the shelf life. Therefore, cakes, cookies, and sweet breads will keep longer than muffins and sandwich breads or dinner rolls. Shelf life may be prolonged by refrigeration, but generally it isn't necessary if you consume the product within the week. I keep cookies in the freezer, not for the sake of keeping them fresh, but for the texture and flavor. Store cakes that have been frosted with *Cream Cheese Frosting*, covered, in either the freezer or refrigerator.

Always refrigerate puddings and pies that contain eggs and milk. Don't leave them on the shelf overnight, or even a few hours. Serious illness could result.

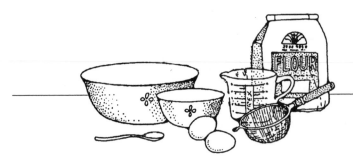

How to Read a Recipe

Recipes in this cookbook are packed with information, some of it technical. However, the format is designed so the important items (e.g. ingredients and procedures) stand out from the details. The example below explains how the data and details relate to the recipe.

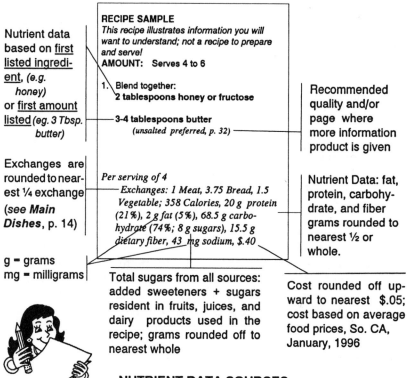

Nutrient data based on <u>first listed ingredient</u>, *(e.g. honey)* or <u>first amount listed</u> *(eg. 3 Tbsp. butter)*

RECIPE SAMPLE
This recipe illustrates information you will want to understand; not a recipe to prepare and serve!
AMOUNT: Serves 4 to 6

1. Blend together:
   2 tablespoons honey or fructose

   3-4 tablespoons butter
   (unsalted preferred, p. 32)

Recommended quality and/or page where more information product is given

Exchanges are rounded to nearest ¼ exchange *(see **Main Dishes**, p. 14)*

Per serving of 4
Exchanges: 1 Meat, 3.75 Bread, 1.5 Vegetable; 358 Calories, 20 g protein (21%), 2 g fat (5%), 68.5 g carbohydrate (74%; 8 g sugars), 15.5 g dietary fiber, 43 mg sodium, $.40

Nutrient Data: fat, protein, carbohydrate, and fiber grams rounded to nearest ½ or whole.

g = grams
mg = milligrams

Total sugars from all sources: added sweeteners + sugars resident in fruits, juices, and dairy products used in the recipe; grams rounded off to nearest whole

Cost rounded off upward to nearest $.05; cost based on average food prices, So. CA, January, 1996

NUTRIENT DATA SOURCES

Nutrient data for this book has been compiled from the following:

Nutrition Wizard, computer data program, Michael Jacobson, Center for Science in the Public Interest, 1986.

Food Values of Portions Commonly Used, *14th Edition*, Jean A.T. Pennington & Helen Nichols Church, Harper & Row, Publishers, 1985.

Nutrition Almanac, *Revised Edition*, Nutrition Search, Inc., John D. Kirschmann, Director, McGraw-Hill Book Company, 1979.

Jean Carper's Total Nutrition Guide, USDA Databases, pp. 222-419, Jean Carper, Bantam Books, 1987.

Laurel's Kitchen, Laurel Robertson, Carol Flinders & Bronwen Godfrey, Nilgiri Press, Berkeley, California, 1976.

Nutrient Facts labels on packaged foods.

Teaching Children

*Train a child in the way he should go
and when he is old he will not turn from it.*
Proverbs 20:6

Can godly parents really determine the course of their children's lives? As adults we do reflect our parents, yet each of us is created with the power to make choices that may lead us into a life path quite different from that of our parents.

Could it be that "*the way he should go*" does not merely refer to the values and standards set by godly parents? It also includes encouraging the child to discover and develop his God-endowed gifts.

Children have a natural interest in food, especially sweets, and in kitchen activities. Take advantange of this interest to teach children not only management skills in food preparation, but nutritional and biblical principles as well. Thus, **Desserts** provides an extension of the *Children's Cookbook* in **Lunches & Snacks**.

Let the **Lunches & Snacks,** *Children's Cookbook*, pp. 33-108, and *What Children Can Learn*, pp. 30-32, be your guide for using **Desserts** for lessons in food preparation, nutrition, and God's purpose for food. *What Children Can Learn* provides guides to what you can expect of children at different ages. Let them get involved. Capture the interest while it is high. You may be introducing the world to another galloping gourmet or even a new frugal gourmet. If your child turns out to be a musician, that's okay. Even musicians have to eat!

Apply some of the research projects (e.g. **Lunches & Snacks**, p. 106) to lessons in making desserts, or design your own research projects. For example, visit the supermarket with your child to make a list of the ingredients in several different packaged desserts and mixes: e.g. ready-made pies, cookies, cake mixes, pudding mixes, etc. Do the same in a health food store. Compare the qualities of ingredients in the two lists, and also with recipes in **Desserts**. Compare prices as well. Have a family discussion about these while eating a favorite dessert around the family table. Such a project can be a real eye-opener as to why we make our own desserts, always aiming for higher nutritional quality.

Another project might be to experiment with ingredient substitutions to develop recipe variations.

Cakes

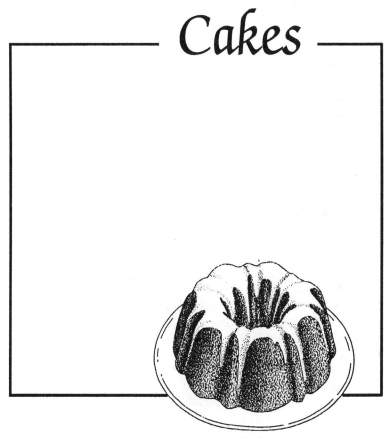

. . . note well what is before you, and put a knife to your throat if you are given to gluttony. . . have the wisdom to show restraint.
Proverbs 23:1-2, 4

Cakes

Angel Food Cake

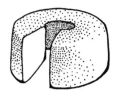

Our son-in-law's favorite cake, deliciously flavorful and moist! Do not expect it to rise as high as the cake mix version with white flour and sugar. Serve plain or topped with fresh berries, whipped cream or topping, ice cream, or Joy's 4-in-1 Non-Dairy Sauce, p. 158.

AMOUNT: Angel Cake Tube Pan (12 - 14 Servings)
Bake 375° for 35-40 minutes

1. Separate <u>about 1½ dozen eggs</u> to make:
   2¼ cups egg whites *(p. 53)*

2. Add and beat with electric mixer on medium speed until frothy:
   2 teaspoons cream of tartar *(p. 15)*
   3/8 teaspoon salt

3. Preheat oven to 375°.

4. Gradually add fructose <u>2 tablespoons at a time</u>
   while beating on high speed:
   1 1/8 cups crystalline fructose *(p. 13)*

5. Continue to beat on high speed until egg whites hold stiff peaks; blend in extracts with just a jog or two with electric beaters:
   4½ teaspoons vanilla extract
   1½ teaspoons almond extract

6. In a separate bowl blend together, stirring ingredients through a strainer (adding the wheat bran left in the strainer):
   1 1/8 cups whole wheat pastry flour *(p. 14)*
   6 tablespoons arrowroot powder *(p. 13)* **or cornstarch**
   ¾ cup crystalline fructose

7. Sprinkle dry ingredients <u>1/3 cup at a time</u> over top of beaten whites and just begin to mix in with a jog or two of electric beaters. After all has been added, gently fold in dry ingredients more evenly with rubber spatula.

8. Gently pile batter into <u>ungreased tube pan</u> and level off; cut through it gently with metal spatula or knife in several places.

9. Bake in center of oven at 375° for 35-40 minutes until golden brown on top and surface feels firm to touch. Invert cake pan to cool thoroughly. Remove cake by carefully loosening it around sides, center post, and bottom with metal spatula.

Per piece of 12
 Exchanges: 0.5 Meat, 0.75 Bread; 206 Calories, 6 g protein (11%), less 1 g fat (1%),
46 g carbohydrate (88%; 31 g sugars), 1.5 g dietary fiber, 0 mg cholesterol, 142 mg sodium, $.55

Applesauce Cupcakes

Delectable with or without frosting. Use a large enough saucepan to mix all the ingredients together in the pan.

AMOUNT: 12 - 15 Cupcakes *(p. 55)*
Bake 350° for 25-30 minutes

1. Preheat oven to 350°. Prepare muffin pan with paper bake cups or grease or spray generously with non-stick spray (pp. 54-55).

2. Melt butter in large saucepan over very low heat; whisk in remaining ingredients one at a time to blend well:
    ½ stick (¼ cup) melted butter *(unsalted preferred, p. 32)*
    ¾ cup honey
    1 egg *(or alternative, p. 39)*
    ¾ cup unsweetened applesauce
    ¼ teaspoon almond extract

3. Blend dry ingredients in mixing bowl:
    2 cups whole wheat pastry flour *(p. 14; or alternative, pp. 20-22)*
    ½ teaspoon cinnamon
    ¼ teaspoon ground cloves
    1½ teaspoons baking powder *(low sodium or Rumford preferred, p. 13)*
    ½ teaspoon baking soda
    ¼ teaspoon salt

4. Whisk dry ingredients into liquid ingredients just until mixed.

5. Fill bake cups 2/3 - ¾ full; bake in preheated oven at 350° for 25-30 minutes. For easier removal cool cupcakes not baked in paper bake cups for 5 minutes before removing from pan.

6. Optional--Frost completely cooled cupcakes with your choice:
    Cream Cheese Frosting   Honey Cream Frosting *(p. 65)*
    Maple Frosting--Variation of *Joy's Non-Dairy Sauce* *(p. 159)*

Per cupcake of 12, unfrosted
  Exchanges: 1 Bread, 0.75 Fat; 195 Calories, 3 g protein (6%), 5 g fat (21%),
38 g carbohydrate (74%; 19 g sugars), 2.5 g dietary fiber, 28 mg cholesterol, 87 mg sodium, $.20

Per cupcake of 12, frosted with Cream Cheese Frosting
  Exchanges: 1 Bread, 3 Fat; 316 Calories, 4.5 g protein (5%), 15 g fat (41%),
45 g carbohydrate (54%; 25 g sugars), 2.5 g dietary fiber, 59 mg cholesterol, 144 mg sodium, $.40

Per cupcake of 12, frosted with Honey Cream Frosting
  Exchanges: 0.25 Milk, 1 Bread, 0.75 Fat; 268 Calories, 6 g protein (9%), 5 g fat (16%),
54 g carbohydrate (76%; 33 g sugars), 2.5 g dietary fiber, 31 mg cholesterol, 129 mg sodium, $.35

Per cupcake of 12, frosted with 2 Tbsps. Maple Frosting
  Exchanges: 1.5 Bread; 1.5 Fat; 267 Calories, 3.5 g protein (5%), 9 g fat (28%),
48 g carbohydrate (67%; 22 g sugars), 3 g dietary fiber, 28 mg cholesterol, 169 mg sodium, $.30

Cream Cheese Frosting

Cream cheese frosting tends to seep slowly into cake. For best results, freeze the cake before frosting it, and frost just before serving. Cover and store leftover cake in refrigerator or freezer (freezer is best).

AMOUNT: Frosts 9" x 13" Cake or 12-18 Cupcakes

Whip cream cheese until soft; blend in remaining ingredients until smooth and creamy:

8 oz. (1 cup) light or *Neufchatel* cream cheese, or cream cheese
½ stick (¼ cup) soft butter *(unsalted preferred, p. 32)*
¼ cup honey
½ teaspoon lemon or orange extract,
**   or 1 teaspoon vanilla extract**
1 teaspoon grated lemon or orange peel, optional
    omit if using vanilla extract *(see Lemon/Orange Peel Tip, p. 106)*

Per Recipe with light cream cheese, vanilla, no lemon or orange peel
*   Exchanges: 22 Fat; 1,248 Calories, 32 g protein (7%), 98 g fat (69%),*
76 g carbohydrate (24%; 75 g sugars), 300 mg cholesterol, 914 mg sodium, $2.25

Honey Cream Frosting

Note that spun honey (available in all supermarkets) is used for this recipe. This is a yummy and very rich frosting, and also very sticky. Use only to frost a cake that will remain in the pan. For cupcakes, make a mound in center of the cupcake, not spreading it to the edges, and top with a nut. Keep frosted cakes refrigerated.

AMOUNT: Frosts 9" x 13" Cake or 12-18 Cupcakes

1. With electric mixer blend thoroughly:
    ½ cup spun honey *(p. 15)*
    2 tablespoons heavy cream or whipping cream
    2 tablespoons soft butter *(unsalted preferred, p. 32)*
    1 teaspoon vanilla

2. Gradually blend in:
    ¾ cup non-instant, nonfat dry milk powder *(p. 14)*
    (stir through a strainer to remove any lumps)

3. Spread on thoroughly cooled cake or cupcakes (see introductory comment above).

Per Recipe
*   Exchanges: 3.5 Milk, 5 Fat; 1,079 Calories, 35 g protein (12%), 27 g fat (21%),*
185 g carbohydrate (67%; 166 g sugars), 92 mg cholesterol, 505 mg sodium, $1.75

Applesauce Cake

A delightfully flavored moist, light cake. When someone requests a whole grain wedding cake recipe, this is the one I suggest (recipe can be multiplied; see p. 80). I make most of my cakes in a bundt pan and serve with a topping. When baked in a 9" x 13" pan I usually frost the cake.

AMOUNT: Bundt Pan or 9" x 13" Pan (24 Servings)
Bake 325° for 50-55 minutes

1. Preheat oven to 325°. Grease or spray bake pan generously with non-stick spray (p. 54).

2. Whisk or beat butter and honey together until well blended; whisk or beat in eggs:
   1½ sticks (¾ cup) butter, melted (unsalted preferred, p. 32)
   1½ cups honey
   3 well beaten eggs (or alternative, p. 39)

3. Blend dry ingredients thoroughly in a separate bowl:
   3 cups whole wheat pastry flour (p. 14; or alternative, pp. 20-22)
   1 teaspoon cinnamon
   ½ teaspoon ground cloves
   2 teaspoons baking powder (low sodium or Rumford preferred, p. 13)
   1½ teaspoons baking soda
   ½ teaspoon salt

4. Thoroughly whisk or beat dry ingredients alternately into liquid ingredients with:
   1½ cups unsweetened applesauce

5. Blend in:
   1 teaspoon almond extract
   1 cup chopped walnuts, optional

6. Pour into greased pan and bake in preheated oven at 325° for 50-55 minutes or until knife comes clean out of center. Cool in pan for 10 minutes before removing.

7. Frost thoroughly cooled cake, or top with one of the following:
   Cream Cheese Frosting (p.65)   *Maple Frosting* (p. 159)
   Honey Vanilla Frosting (p. 69)   *Lemon Sauce* (p. 155)
   Whipped Cream/Topping (pp. 155, 159)   *Pineapple Topping* (p. 157)

Per piece of 24 <u>without nuts, unfrosted</u>
(bundt pan cut 1 piece per narrow scallop, 2 pieces per wide scallop)
   Exchanges: 1 Bread, 1 Fat; 190 Calories, 2.5 g protein (5%), 7 g fat (30%),
33 g carbohydrate (65%; 19 g sugars), 2 g dietary fiber, 42 mg cholesterol, 107 mg sodium, $.20

Per piece of 24 <u>with nuts, frosted with Cream Cheese Frosting</u> (9" x 13" pan cut 6 x 4)
   Exchanges: 1 Bread, 2.5 Fat; 250 Calories, 3.5 g protein (5%), 12 g fat (41%),
58 g carbohydrate (54%; 22 g sugars), 2 g dietary fiber, 58 mg cholesterol, 135 mg sodium, $.30

Carrot Cake

Light, tender, moist, and not too sweet. For a rich dessert cake, this is our favorite. Our girls made this, frosted with Cream Cheese Frosting for our 25th Wedding Anniversary. Before starting step #1 grate the carrots, drain the pineapple, chop the nuts, measure the raisins.

AMOUNT: 9" x 13" Pan or Bundt Pan (24 Servings)
Bake 325° for 45-55 minutes

1. Preheat oven to 325°. Grease or spray bake pan generously with non-stick spray (p. 54).

2. In large mixing bowl whisk or beat butter and honey together until well blended; whisk or beat in remaining ingredients:
   - **1 stick (½ cup) butter, melted** *(unsalted preferred, p. 32)*
   - **¾ cup honey**
   - **4 eggs** *(or alternative, p. 39)*
   - **1 teaspoon vanilla**
   - **3 cups shredded carrot**
   - **1-1¼ cups crushed pineapple, drained** (from 20 oz. can)

3. Blend dry ingredients thoroughly in a separate bowl:
   - **2½ cups whole wheat pastry flour** *(p. 14; or alternative, pp. 20-22)*
   - **1 teaspoon cinnamon**
   - **2 teaspoons baking soda**
   - **¾ teaspoon salt**

4. Thoroughly whisk or beat dry ingredients into liquid ingredients; fold in:
   - **1 cup chopped walnuts**
   - **1 cup raisins, optional**

5. Pour into greased pan. Bake in preheated oven at 325° for 45-55 minutes or until a knife comes clean out of center. Cool in pan for 10 minutes before removing.

6. Cool thoroughly and frost or top with one of the following:
   - *Cream Cheese Frosting* (p. 65)
   - *Whipped Cream* or *Whipped Topping* (pp. 155, 159)

Per piece of 24 with raisins, <u>unfrosted</u>
(bundt pan cut 1 piece per narrow scallop, 2 pieces per wide scallop)
   Exchanges: 0.25 Meat, 0.75 Bread, 1.25 Fat, 0.5 Fruit, 0.25 Vegetable; 196 Calories, 4 g protein (8%), 8 g fat (35%), 30 g carbohydrate (57%; 16 g sugars), 3 g dietary fiber, 46 mg cholesterol, 162 mg sodium, $.25

Per piece of 24 with raisins, <u>frosted with Cream Cheese Frosting</u> (9" x 13" pan cut 6 x 4)
   Exchanges: 0.25 Meat, 0.75 Bread, 2.5 Fat, 0.5 Fruit, 0.25 Vegetable; 254 Calories, 5 g protein (7%), 13 g fat (44%), 33 g carbohydrate (48%; 19 g sugars), 2.5 g dietary fiber, 61 mg cholesterol, 182 mg sodium, $.35

Chocolate Cupcakes

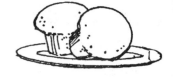

Great for child's party, or snack treat.

AMOUNT: 12 - 15 Cupcakes *(p. 55)*
Bake 350° for 25-30 minutes

1. Preheat oven to 350°. Prepare muffin pan with paper bake cups or grease or spray generously with non-stick spray (pp. 54-55).

2. Melt butter and chocolate over very low heat in large saucepan that will hold all the ingredients; whisk in remaining ingredients:
    ½ stick (¼ cup) butter *(unsalted preferred, p. 32)*
    1 oz. square unsweetened chocolate
    ¼ cup hot water
    ¾ cup honey
    2 eggs *(or alternative, p. 39)*
    ½ cup buttermilk *(or alternative, p. 39)*
    1 teaspoon vanilla

3. Blend dry ingredients in mixing bowl:
    1 2/3 cups whole wheat pastry flour *(p. 14; or alternative, pp. 20-22)*
    ¼ cup cocoa powder (stir through strainer to remove lumps)
    1 teaspoon baking soda
    ½ teaspoon baking powder *(low sodium or Rumford preferred, p. 13)*
    ½ teaspoon salt

4. Whisk dry ingredients into liquid ingredients just until mixed.

5. Fold in:
    ½ cup chopped walnuts, optional

6. Fill cups 2/3 - ¾ full; bake in preheated oven at 350° for 25-30 minutes. For easier removal cool cupcakes not baked in paper bake cups for 5 minutes before removing from pan.

7. Frost completely cooled cupcakes with:
    Chocolate Frosting or Honey Vanilla Frosting, *(p. 69)*

Per cupcake of 12 without walnuts, frosted with Chocolate Frosting
    Exchanges: 0.25 Meat, 1 Bread, 2.75 Fat; 300 Calories, 5 g protein (7%), 15 g fat (42%), 40 g carbohydrate (51%; 23 g sugars), mg cholesterol, mg. sodium $.35

Carob Cupcakes

Increase water to **6 tablespoons hot water**. Replace chocolate and cocoa with **scant ½ cup carob powder** *(p. 13)*. Frost with *Carob Frosting* *(p. 69)*.

Per cupcake of 12 without walnuts, frosted with Carob Frosting
    Exchanges: 0.25 Meat, 1.5 Bread, 2.5 Fat; 302 Calories, 4.5 g protein (6%), 13 g fat (38%), 45 g carbohydrate (57%; 19 g sugars), 2.5 g dietary fiber, 84 mg cholesterol, 190 mg sodium, $.35

Carob or Chocolate Frosting

A delectably rich frosting. Triple the recipe for a 2-layer cake.

AMOUNT: Frosts 9" x 13" Cake or 12-18 Cupcakes

1. Blend in electric mixer until light and creamy:
   1 stick (½ cup) soft butter *(unsalted preferred, p. 32)*
   ¼ cup crystalline fructose *(p. 13)* **or mild-flavored honey** *(p. 25)*

2. Blend in until creamy and spreadable:
   1 egg *(or alternative, p. 39)*
   ¼ cup carob powder *(p. 13)* **or cooca powder**
   (stir through a strainer to remove lumps)
   1 teaspoon vanilla
   optional: 1 tablespoon crystalline fructose or honey, to taste
   (to increase sweetness, if desired)

3. Spread on thoroughly cooled cake or cupcakes.

Per <u>Carob</u> Frosting Recipe, optional sweetening not included
  Exchanges: 1 Meat, 1.75 Bread, 18.5 Fat; 1,185 Calories, 8.5 g protein (3%), 96 g fat (71%),
  79 g carbohydrate (26%; 50 g sugars), 2.5 g dietary fiber, 461 mg cholesterol, 87 mg sodium, $1.25

Per <u>Chocolate</u> Frosting Recipe, optional sweetening not included
  Exchanges: 1.25 Meat, 0.5 Bread, 19 Fat; 1,158 Calories, 13 g protein (4%), 99 g fat (75%),
  60 g carbohydrate (20%; 50 g sugars), 1 g dietary fiber, 461 mg cholesterol, 86 mg sodium, $1.40

Honey Vanilla Frosting

A totally nonfat frosting!

AMOUNT: Frosts 8" or 9" Square Cake or 12 Cupcakes

1. Beat with electric mixer until peaks are formed:
   1 egg white *(p. 53)*
   ¼ teaspoon cream of tartar *(p. 15)*
   1/8 teaspoon salt

2. Pour honey in slow stream into egg white
   while continuing to beat; add vanilla:
   ½ cup honey
   1 teaspoon vanilla

3. Continue beating about 5-10 minutes longer, or until
   of spreadable consistency that will not drip off cake.

4. Mound on cupcakes or cake with spoon and use the back of the
   spoon to spread evenly over the top. Refrigerate Cake.

Per Recipe
  Exchanges: 0.25 Meat; 530 Calories, 3.5 g protein (3%),
  239 g carbohydrate (98%; 138 g sugars), 0 mg cholesterol, 325 mg sodium, $.95

Chocolate or Carob Cake

Moist and tender, this cake is a pleasing blend of subtle chocolate or carob, and dates. No frosting needed, but for a rich chocolate or carob flavor, frost with Chocolate or Carob Frosting, p. 69.

AMOUNT: 9" x 13" Pan or Bundt Pan (24 Servings)
Bake 325° for 30-40 Minutes

1. Preheat oven to 325°. Grease or spray bake pan generously with non-stick spray (p. 54).

2. Pour water over dates; whisk in soda:
   ¾ cup date dices or nuggets *(p. 13)* **or chopped dates** *(see tip, p. 71)*
   ¾ cup boiling hot water
   1½ teaspoons baking soda

3. In a separate large bowl whisk or beat together until smooth and creamy:
   1 1/8 cups honey
   1½ cups mayonnaise *(see Shopping Tip below)*
   1½ teaspoons vanilla

4. Whisk or beat date mixture into honey mixture to blend well.

5. Blend dry ingredients together in separate bowl:
   2 5/8 cups whole wheat pastry flour *(p. 14; or alternative, pp. 20-22)*
   6 tablespoons cocoa powder or carob powder *(p. 13)*
   (stir through strainer to remove lumps)
   1½ teaspoons cinnamon
   3/8 teaspoon salt

6. Thoroughly whisk or beat dry ingredients into liquid ingredients; fold in:
   1 cup walnuts, chopped, optional

7. Pour into greased pan and bake in preheated oven at 325° for 30-40 minutes or until knife comes clean out of center.

Per piece of 24, <u>Unfrosted</u> Chocolate or Carob Cake; without nuts
(cut 9" x 13" pan 6 x 4 or bundt pan 1 piece per narrow scallop, 2 pieces per wide scallop)
*   Exchanges: 0.75 Bread, 2.5 Fat, 0.25 Fruit; 234 Calories, 2 g protein (3-4%), 12.5 g fat (46%),*
31 g carbohydrate (50-51%; 16 g sugars), 2 g dietary fiber, 5 mg cholesterol, 166 mg sodium, $.20

Per piece of 24, <u>Frosted</u> Chocolate or Carob Cake; without nuts
(cut 9" x 13" pan 6 x 4 or bundt pan 1 piece per narrow scallop, 2 pieces per wide scallop)
*   Exchanges: 1 Bread, 3.25 Fat, 0.25 Fruit; 284 Calories, 2.5 g protein (3%), 16.5 g fat (50-51%),*
34 g carbohydrate (45-47%; 16 g sugars), 2 g dietary fiber, 24 mg cholesterol, 170 mg sodium, $.25

Mayonnaise Shopping Tip: *Hollywood* brand mayonnaise at supermarkets and *Hain* brand at health food stores contain no refined sugar or preservatives.

Date Nut Cake

A rich flavorful moist cake that needs no frosting.

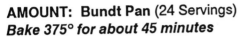

AMOUNT: Bundt Pan (24 Servings)
Bake 375° for about 45 minutes

1. Preheat oven to 325°. Grease or spray bake pan generously with non-stick spray (p. 54).

2. Whisk or beat together until well blended:
   1½ sticks (¾ cup) butter, melted *(unsalted preferred, p. 32)*
   ¾ cup honey

3. Whisk together and blend into butter-honey:
   5 small ripe bananas, mashed
   4 large or 5 medium well-beaten eggs *(or alternative, p. 39)*
   4½ teaspoons water
   3 teaspoons vanilla

4. Blend dry ingredients thoroughly in a separate bowl:
   1 3/8 cups whole wheat pastry flour *(p. 14; or alternative, pp. 20-22)*
   ½ cup arrowroot powder *(p. 44)* **or whole wheat pastry flour**
   3 teaspoons baking soda
   1½ teaspoons salt

5. Whisk or beat dry ingredients into liquid ingredients; Fold in:
   ¾ cup chopped walnuts
   ¾ cup chopped date dices or nuggets or dates *(p. 13; see tip below)*

6. Pour into greased pan. Bake in preheated oven at 375° for about 45 minutes or until a knife comes clean out of center.

7. Cool in pan for 10 minutes before removing.

Per piece of 24 (bundt pan cut 1 piece per narrow scallop, 2 pieces per wide scallop)
  Exchanges: 0.5 Bread, 1.5 Fat, 0.5 Fruit; 192 Calories, 3.5 g protein (7%), 9 g fat (40%), 27 g carbohydrate (53%; 17 g sugars), 2 g dietary fiber, 51 mg cholesterol, 249 mg sodium, $.30

Dried Fruit Chopping Tip: Cut dried fruits into pieces, such as pitted dates and figs, with kitchen shears. Cut dates in half lengthwise, then the two halves together crosswise into small pieces. Cut figs lengthwise into 3 or 4 pieces, then together crosswise in small pieces. If recipe calls for it, chop date dices or nuggets with with a chef's knife (p.49).

German Chocolate Cake

*A yummy rich gourmet cake! Plan on getting at least 16
servings out of this. Michael J. Phillips, novelist and
editor of the Bethany House George McDonald novels,
enjoys it on his birthday, with slight modifications, lovingly baked by his
wife, Judy. Give yourself plenty of leisure time to make this cake. Toast the
almonds, if needed, and prepare filling, p. 73, a few hours in advance.*

AMOUNT: Triple 9" Layer Cake
Bake 350° for 25-30 Minutes

1. Make the **Filling**, p. 73, and set aside to cool thoroughly, but
   for ease of spreading do not allow it to firm up too much.

2. Grease or spray 3 - 9" round layer cake pans. Cut circles
   of wax paper to fit bottoms of pans (p. 54); place paper in
   pans and lightly grease or spray again. Preheat oven to 350°.

3. In saucepan place over very low heat until chocolate melts:
   1 cup water
   3 squares unsweetened chocolate

4. In large mixing bowl, whisk or beat butter and honey together
   until well blended and smooth; blend in vanilla and egg whites;
   1½ sticks (¾ cup) soft butter *(unsalted preferred, p. 32)*
   1¾ cups honey
   1½ teaspoons vanilla
   separated egg whites, unbeaten

5. Blend dry ingredients in separate bowl:
   2½ cups whole wheat pastry flour *(p. 14; or alternative, pp. 20-22)*
   ½ cup arrowroot powder *(p. 44)*
   2¼ teaspoons baking soda
   ¾ teaspoon salt

6. Alternately blend dry ingredients and melted chocolate
   into honey-butter mixture beginning and ending with dry
   ingredients.

7. Pour batter evenly into prepared layer cake pans and bake
   in preheated oven at 350° for 25-30 minutes or until knife comes
   clean out of center. Allow to cool 10 minutes before removing
   from pans; cool layers on cake rack. Remove wax paper.

8. Evenly spread **Filling** between completely cooled layers
   on large serving plate; Frost sides and top with **Frosting**, p.73.

9. Store cake in freezer until ½ hour before serving. Refrigerator
   is okay for a short time if freezer space is not available.

FILLING (for German Chocolate Cake)

1. Separate **6 eggs**, placing yolks and whites in separate bowls.

2. Heat together in large saucepan over moderately low heat:
   1 cup nonfat milk *(or alternative, p. 39)*
   ½ cup honey

3. Gradually whisk a small amount of hot milk mixture into
   separated egg yolks; whisk back into milk mixture remaining
   in sauce pan. Continue to cook over moderate heat, whisking constantly until lightly thickened.

4. Remove from heat and thoroughly blend in remaining
   ingredients; set aside to cool:
   ½ stick (¼ cup) butter *(unsalted preferred, p. 32)*
   1 teaspoon vanilla
   2 cups unsweetened coconut, medium shred *(p. 13)*
   1½ cups whole toasted almonds, chopped *(see below)*

> **Toasted Almonds:** The toasted almonds are essential to the flavor of this cake.
> Purchase roasted, unsalted, at a health food store, or toast whole raw almonds
> in single layer in a shallow pan in 300° oven to desired doneness, about 20-
> 30 minutes; stir occasionally.   Cool; chop with chef's knife (p. 49).

German Chocolate Cake Frosting

*A sumptuous amount of light fluffy frosting! Good for other chocolate
cakes too (should be kept in the freezer).*

1. Gradually add remaining ingredients to whipping cream while
   whipping at high speed with electric mixer until whipped:
   2 cups (1 pint) whipping cream *(raw certified preferred, p. 39)*
   6 tablespoons crystalline fructose *(p. 13),*
   (stir through strainer to remove any lumps)
   ¼ cup cocoa powder (stir through strainer)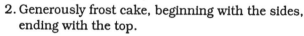
   1 teaspoon vanilla

2. Generously frost cake, beginning with the sides,
   ending with the top.

> **Frosting Layer Cake Tip:** Place a mound of frosting on top of cake near the
> edge; with metal spatula or table knife, gently spread over the edge and down
> the side of cake; repeat around the cake to finish sides; then frost the top.

Per piece of 16, filled and frosted
   Exchanges: 0.75 Meat, 1.5 Bread, 7 Fat; 655 Calories, 10 g protein (6%),
40 g fat (52%), 73 g carbohydrate (42%; 44 g sugars), 5.5 g dietary fiber, 152 mg cholesterol,
261 mg sodium, $.80

Gingerbread Cake

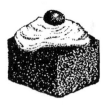

Serve with warm applesauce or whipped cream. Choose light or mild, dark, or blackstrap molasses depending on how strong a molasses flavor is pleasing to your taste (p. 27).

AMOUNT: 9" Square Bake Pan (9-12 Servings)
Bake 325° for 50-55 minutes

1. Preheat oven to 325°. Grease or spray bake pan with non-stick spray (p. 54).

2. Whisk together to blend thoroughly:
   1 stick (½ cup) soft butter *(unsalted preferred, p. 32)*
   ¾ cup honey
   1 egg *(or alternative, p. 39)*
   ½ cup molasses *(p. 27)*

3. Blend dry ingredients thoroughly in a separate bowl:
   2½ cups whole wheat pastry flour *(p. 14; or alternative, pp. 20-22)*
   1 teaspoon cinnamon
   1 teaspoon ground ginger
   ½ teaspoon ground cloves
   2 teaspoons baking powder *(low sodium or Rumford preferred, p. 13)*
   ½ teaspoon salt

4. Whisk dry ingredients into liquid ingredients. Whisk into batter until well blended:
   1 cup hot water

5. Pour into pan (batter will be soupy). Bake in preheated 325° oven for about 50-55 minutes until knife comes clean out of center.

Per serving of 9 (pan cut 3 x 3) with blackstrap molasses
   Exchanges: 2 Bread, 2 Fat; 363 Calories, 5 g protein (5%), 11.5 g fat (27%), 66 g carbohydrate (68%; 35 g sugars), 4 g dietary fiber, 51 mg cholesterol, 149 mg sodium, $.35

Per serving of 12 (pan cut 3 x 4) with blackstrap molasses
   Exchanges: 1.5 Bread, 1.5 Fat; 272 Calories, 3.5 g protein (5%), 8.5 g fat (27%), 49 g carbohydrate (68%; 26 g sugars), 3 g dietary fiber 38 mg cholesterol, 112 mg sodium, $.25

VARIATION

Can be baked at 350° for about 30 minutes, if desired.

Orange Chiffon Cake

A light cake with a sweet orange glaze with half the fat of the original.

AMOUNT: Angel Cake Tube Pan (12 - 14 Servings)
Bake 350° for 45-50 minutes

1. Separate **6 large eggs** (p. 53). Allow whites to come to room temperature.

2. Preheat oven to 350°.

3. In a medium mixing bowl evenly blend dry ingredients:
   2 cups whole wheat pastry flour *(p. 14)*
   1 cup crystalline fructose *(p. 13)*
   4 teaspoons baking powder *(low sodium or Rumford preferred, p. 13)*
   1 teaspoon salt

4. In large mixing bowl whisk first three ingredients thoroughly; whisk in dry ingredients until smooth, about 1-2 minutes:
   6 egg yolks
   ¾ cup fresh orange juice
   2 tablespoons grated orange peel
   dry ingredients (#3 above)

5. Beat egg whites on high speed with electric mixer until stiff enough to hold peaks, but not dry (p. 54):
   6 egg whites
   ½ teaspoon cream of tartar *(p. 15)*

6. Gently fold stiffly beaten egg whites into batter until evenly blended. Pile batter evenly into ungreased tube cake pan; Bake at 350° for 45-60 minutes or until toothpick comes clean out of center. Invert cake pan to cool thoroughly.

7. Remove cake by carefully loosening it around sides, post, and bottom with metal spatula. Frost top, then sides with glaze.

8. For **Glaze**, whisk together:
   ½ stick (¼ cup) melted butter
   1 cup crystalline fructose*
   3 tablespoons orange juice
   1 - 3 teaspoons grated orange peel

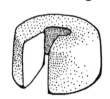

Per piece of 12   Exchanges: 0.5 Meat, 1.25 Bread, 1 Fat; 0.25 Fruit; 296 Calories, 5.5 g protein (7%), 7 g fat (21%), 55 g carbohydrate (72%; 39 g sugars), 2.5 g dietary fiber, 117 mg cholesterol, 252 mg sodium, $.35

*If desired, for a powdered sugar texture, powder the fructose in a blender, blending half of it at a time. If fructose is lumpy, stir it through a strainer to remove all lumps before powdering it in blender.

No-Bake Honey Cheese Cake

A delectable cheesecake, yet lower in calories and fat than most, and requires no baking! This recipe has a light graham cracker crumb topping and no crust. To make it with a crust, use the crust recipe for Yogurt Pie, p. 128. In place of crumb mixture topping, use fresh strawberries or Strawberry Topping, p. 158, or garnish cake with other fresh fruit.

AMOUNT: 8"-9" Square Pan (About 9 Servings)

1. In small saucepan whisk gelatine into water; let stand 5 minutes to soften; heat to boiling while stirring with whisk until gelatine is dissolved:
   ¼ cup cold water (room temperature)
   1 envelope (2 teaspoons) unflavored gelatine *(p. 45)*

2. In blender, blend together until smooth in order given:
   1 egg
   1/3 cup mild-flavored honey *(p. 25)*
   1 teaspoon vanilla
   8 oz. (1 cup) cream cheese or light cream cheese, softened (add gradually in small pieces)
   ½ cup lowfat or nonfat plain yogurt *(or pasteurized alternative, p. 39)*
   ½ cup sour cream or light sour cream
   dissolved gelatine

3. Pour mixture into 8"-9" square pan; chill until set.

4. For graham cracker topping blend together:
   ¼ cup graham cracker crumbs *(p. 13; see tip, p. 119)*
   1 tablespoon crystalline fructose *(p. 13)*
   or 2 tablespoons sugar
   1 tablespoon melted butter *(unsalted preferred, p. 32)*

5. Sprinkle crumb topping over cheesecake anytime during chilling process or just before serving.

Per serving of 9 <u>*with cream cheese, lowfat yogurt, sour cream*</u>
   Exchanges: 0.25 Meat, 0.25 Milk, 0.25 Bread, 2.75 Fat; 201 Calories, 4.5 g protein (9%), 14 g fat (61%), 16 g carbohydrate (31%; 13 g sugars), 61 mg cholesterol, 121 mg sodium, $.35

Per serving of 9 <u>*with light cream cheese, nonfat yogurt, light sour cream*</u>
   Exchanges: 0.25 Meat, 0.25 Milk, 0.25 Bread, 2 Fat; 168 Calories, 5.5 g protein (13%), 9 g fat (50%), 16 g carbohydrate (37%; 13 g sugars), 51 mg cholesterol, 149 mg sodium, $.40

Per serving of 9 <u>*with light cream cheese, nonfat yogurt, light sour cream, graham cracker crust*</u>
   Exchanges: 0.25 Meat, 0.25 Milk, 0.75 Bread, 2.75 Fat; 236 Calories, 6 g protein (10%), 13.5 g fat (53%), 21 g carbohydrate (37%; 14 g sugars), 0.5 g dietary fiber, 62 mg cholesterol, 215 mg sodium, $.45

Pineapple Up-Side-Down Cake

One of my childhood favorites Mother made often. Serve, if desired, with whipped cream or topping.

AMOUNT: 9" Square Bake Pan (9 Servings)
Bake 350° for 30 minutes

1. Preheat oven to 350°. Grease or spray bake pan generously with non-stick spray (p. 54).

2. Stir fructose and pecans into butter just to combine (do not overmix or mixture will separate); pat evenly with spoon in bottom of bake pan:
   ½ stick (¼ cup) butter, melted *(unsalted preferred, p. 32)*
   (melt an **extra 1 Tbsp.** and set aside to add to egg yolks in step #4)
   ½ cup crystalline fructose *(p. 13)*
   ½ cup chopped pecans

3. Cut pineapple slices in half; arrange over topping mixture:
   6 slices canned pineapple unsweetened, drained
   (1½ - 8 oz. cans)

4. Separate **4 eggs** (p. 53); whisk together thoroughly in large mixing bowl: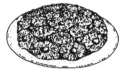
   4 egg yolks *(or alternative, p. 39)*
   1 tablespoon melted butter
   1 teaspoon vanilla

5. Beat egg whites until stiff, but not dry, folding fructose in gradually when eggs reach foamy stage; fold into egg yolk mixture:
   4 egg whites
   2/3 cup crystalline fructose

6. Blend dry ingredients thoroughly; fold carefully, ¼ cup at a time into egg mixture:
   1 cup whole wheat pastry flour *(p. 14; or alternative, pp. 20-22)*
   1 teaspoon baking powder *(low sodium or Rumford preferred, p. 13)*
   ¼ teaspoon salt

7. Spread batter over pineapple slices in bake pan; bake in preheated 350° oven for 30 minutes.

8. Turn cake immediately out on serving plate; leave pan over cake a couple minutes to allow topping to drip over it.

Per piece of 9, cut 3 x 3
   Exchanges: 0.5 Meat, 0.75 Bread, 1.75 Fat, 0.25 Fruit; 282 Calories, 5 g protein (7%), 11 g fat (33%), 44 g carbohydrate (60%; 29 g sugars), 2.5 g dietary fiber, 103 mg cholesterol, 91 mg sodium, $.45

Poppy Seed Cake

Our son Dan's favorite cake.

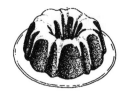

AMOUNT: Bundt Pan (24 Servings)
Bake 325° for 60-65 Minutes

1. Preheat oven to 325°. Grease or spray bake pan generously with non-stick spray (p. 54).

2. In large mixing bowl whisk or beat together thoroughly until light and creamy:
   1 stick (½ cup) soft butter *(unsalted preferred, p. 32)*
   1½ cups honey
   1 teaspoon vanilla

3. Whisk or beat in well, one at a time:
   4 eggs *(or alternative, p. 39)*

4. Whisk together in a measuring cup and set aside:
   ½ cup buttermilk, or yogurt (thinned to buttermilk consistency)
   (or non-dairy alternative soured with ½ Tbsp. vinegar, p. 39)
   1/3 - ½ cup mashed banana (1 medium banana)

5. Blend dry ingredients together in separate bowl:
   3 cups whole wheat pastry flour *(p. 14; or alternative, pp. 20-22)*
   1/3 cup poppy seeds *(p. 15)*
   2½ teaspoons baking soda

6. Alternately whisk or beat dry ingredients and banana-buttermilk mixture into honey-butter, until well mixed after each addition.

7. Pour into greased pan and bake in preheated oven at 325° for 60-65 minutes or until knife comes clean out of center. Cool 10 minutes before removing from pan.

8. Serve plain or top with one of the following:
   Lemon Sauce *(p. 155)*
   Pineapple Topping *(p. 157)*
   Whipped Cream or Whipped Topping *(pp. 155, 159)*
   Honey Vanilla Ice Cream *(p. 141)*
   Frozen Vanilla Yogurt *(p. 141)*

Per piece of 24 (bundt pan cut 1 piece per narrow scallop, 2 pieces per wide scallop)
  Exchanges: 0.25 Meat, 1 Bread, 1 Fat; 189 Calories, 3.5 g protein (7%), 6 g fat (27%),
34 g carbohydrate (66%; 19 g sugars), 2 g dietary fiber, 46 mg cholesterol, 105 mg sodium, $.25

Scripture Fruit Cake

See how well you can translate this nutty fruit cake by looking up the Bible verses before consulting the interpretation below. For time efficiency, prepare items in steps #1, 6, and set out Judges 5:25 the night before.

AMOUNT: 2 Medium or 6 Mini Loaf Pans *(p. 47)*
Bake 300° for 80-90 minutes

1. Grease or spray bake pans with non-stick spray. Line bottoms of pans with wax paper (p. 54); spray paper lightly with non-stick spray.

2. Preheat oven to 300°.

3. In large mixing bowl whisk together the *Judges*, *Proverbs*, and *Jeremiah* until mixed; whisk in *Luke 11:12* to blend well:
   ½ **very soft *Judges 5:25*** *(last food listed, King James Version)*
   2 tablespoons *Proverbs 25:16*
   2 cups *Jeremiah 6:20* (add gradually)*(use the whole kind, see p. 26)*
   8 large *Luke 11:12*, well beaten *(or alternative, p. 39)*

4. Blend together in a separate bowl:
   1½ cups *1 Kings 17:14* *(NIV or NASB, 1st listed food item, whole, see p. 19)*
   2 teaspoons *Matthew 13:33* *(kind used in quick breads, see p. 44)*
   4 teaspoons *2 Chronicles 9:9* *(specific interpretation below)*
   1/8 teaspoon *Matthew 5:13*

5. Blend dry ingredients into liquid ingredients alternately with:
   ½ cup *Hebrews 5:12* *(first food listed, or alternative, p. 39)*

6. Stir in until evenly mixed:
   2 cups (12 oz. pkg.) chopped *Genesis 43:11* *(last food listed)*
   2 cups chopped *2 Kings 20:7* *(p. 15; preparation tip, p. 71)*
   2 Cups *1 Samuel 30:12* *(2nd food listed)*

7. Evenly divide batter in pans and bake in preheated oven at 300° for 80-90 minutes or until a toothpick or knife comes clean out of center.

8. Loosen cake from sides of pans with knife, if necessary; remove from pans, remove wax paper, and cool on side.

Per slice (16 per medium loaf)   Exchanges: 0.5 Meat, 0.5 Bread, 1.5 Fruit; 233 Calories, 5 g protein (8%), 9.5 g fat (34%), 61 g carbohydrate (58%; 22 g sugars), 3.5 g dietary fiber, 61 mg cholesterol, 31 mg sodium, $.40

Interpretation: Luke 11:12 - eggs, large; Judges 5:25 - butter, unsalted preferred
Jeremiah 6:20 - *Sucanat*; Proverbs 25:16 - honey; 1 Kings 17:24 - whole wheat pastry flour
Matthew 13:33 - baking powder, low sodium or Rumford preferred
2 Chronicles 9:9 - 2 tsps. cinnamon, 1 tsp. nutmeg, ½ tsp. ginger, ½ tsp. ground cloves
Matthew 5:13 - salt; Hebrews 5:12 - milk, nonfat
Genesis 43:11 - almonds; 2 Kings 20:7 - figs, unsulfured dried black; 1 Samuel 30:12 - raisins

The Making of Three Cakes

My First Wedding Cake

I had never decorated a wedding cake. Yet my roommate and I warmly agreed to Linda's request that we do the cake for her August wedding. Summer school studies at the University of Washington pressed me for time, so there was no opportunity to practice. Finally a week before the wedding we thought we should practice a few decorating techniques. First, we discovered that our oven wouldn't hold pans large enough for a 3-tiered cake for 225 people. We put in an order to a bakery. A sensible bride would do that, but doing it yourself was something of a tradition. We started putting on borders that slipped and rose cascades that wilted. We commiserated and prayed for miracles. By the early morning hours the cake began to appear beautiful, even "original." Balancing it in the back seat of the car on the way to the church was another peril, but the cake survived. Twenty-six years later Linda did invite me to her daughter's wedding. She made no mention of cakes. I didn't volunteer either.

A Healthy Wedding Cake

Barbara, my globe-trotting friend who long ago learned hard lessons about the consequences of poor food choices, wanted a "healthy" wedding cake. Much wiser now, I consulted a cake decorating friend who agreed to bake my *Applesauce Cake*. 250 guests enjoyed a professionally decorated and delicious freshly ground whole wheat pastry flour cake. I persuaded Barbara to forego a healthy frosting (i.e *Cream Cheese Frosting*) because it would probably slide off the sides as the reception room got warmer and warmer. I consoled her that she would only have to serve "junk" frosting just once and that it was all right to scrape it off her piece after the first bite.

A Birthday Cake

My 8 and 3 year old daughters perched on stool and chair looking on as I finished frosting a traditional Jesus' Birthday Cake. That was before I knew anything other than white flour-white sugar cakes. The girls wanted to put the M&M's on but I doubted that they could neatly spell out "Happy Birthday Jesus" so I put them off. With the decorating completed we persuaded Dad to get the camera. The perfect picture would have mom holding the cake while two bright-eyed girls looked on. Instead, the cake slipped out of my hand landing the frosted top against the kitchen wall. The picture revealed a tearful 8 year old and a very sad 3 year old with a chagrined mother who learned a lesson. From that time on I always invited eager and handy children to make and decorate cakes. Now we make a whole wheat *Angel Food Cake*, p.63, and omit the M&M's (see **Holiday Menus**, p. 45, for Jesus' birthday cake decorating ideas).

Cookies
& Candies

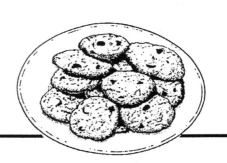

The rod of correction imparts wisdom,
but a child left to itself disgraces his mother.
Proverbs 29:15
Don't let him raid the cookie jar without permission!

Cookies & Candies

CANDIES

COOKIES

*Rolled cookies need not be rolled if shaped with a scoop dispenser (see p. 55)

Almond Roca

Not the same shape as its commercial counterpart, but with the same yummy taste! Use unsalted butter in this recipe if you wish. I prefer that "extra something" in the flavor imparted by lightly salted butter.

AMOUNT: About 1¾ lbs. (About 28 - 1 oz. Pieces)

1. Generously butter a cookie sheet or 13" round pizza pan.

2. Prepare and set aside:
   ½ cup whole almonds, crushed (crush in blender)
   1 cup whole almonds, chopped (not as fine as crushed almonds but fairly well chopped--a chef's knife works well for this)
   1 cup chocolate or carob chips(place in glass measuring cup) *(p. 13)*

3. Whisk together in saucepan until well blended:
   2 sticks (1 cup) lightly salted butter, melted
   1 cup honey

4. Attach candy thermometer to saucepan so that bulb is suspended in ingredients without touching the bottom. Bring to a boil over moderate heat, watching carefully so it does not boil over. Keep boiling steadily, but moderately, until temperature reaches 270° (soft crack stage). This takes about 20-25 minutes. Do not stir during this time.

5. As soon as the thermometer hits 270° (do not let it go over), immediately remove saucepan from heat, add **crushed almonds** and whisk to thoroughly reblend honey and butter until mixture turns creamy and amber in color.

6. Pour candy mixture evenly onto buttered pan, tilting it to spread candy out as far as it will go. Cool while melting the chips.

7. Melt the **chocolate or carob chips** in glass measuring cup set in a pan of hot water over moderately low heat.

8. Spread **melted chocolate or carob** evenly over the top of candy; sprinkle **chopped almonds** evenly over top of chocolate or carob, pressing them into it.

9. Store in freezer. Break off pieces to eat like peanut brittle; a chef's knife works perfectly for this.

Per 1 oz. piece (about 2" square), with chocolate chips
   Exchanges: 2.5 Fat; 170 Calories, 1.5 g protein (4%), 12.5 g fat (63%),
15 g carbohydrate (33%; 14 g sugars), 0.5 g dietary fiber, 18 mg cholesterol, 68 mg sodium, $.20

Per 1 oz. piece (about 2" square), with unsweetened carob chips
   Exchanges: 0.25 Bread, 2.25 Fat; 170 Calories, 2 g protein (5%), 12 g fat (61%),
15 g carbohydrate (34%; 10 g sugars), 0.5 g dietary fiber, 18 mg cholesterol, 67 mg sodium, $.20

Almond Tea Cakes

These delicate crunchy cookies will just melt in your mouth!

AMOUNT: About 2 Dozen
Bake 350° for 12-15 minutes

1. Whisk until soft:
   1 stick (½ cup) soft butter *(unsalted preferred, p. 32)*

2. Blend in thoroughly:
   ¼ cup crystalline fructose *(p. 13)*
   3 teaspoons vanilla
   1/8 teaspoon salt
   1½ cups whole wheat pastry flour *(p. 14; or alternative, pp. 20-22)*
   1 cup finely chopped almonds (can do in blender)

3. Chill dough in refrigerator for 30 minutes, if needed
   for easy handling.

4. Preheat oven to 350°.

5. Roll tablespoons of dough in palms of hands or dispense
   with all-purpose scoop (p. 48) onto ungreased cookie sheet.
   Leave 2" between cookies.

6. Bake 12-15 minutes until golden brown.

7. Allow to cool a bit before removing from cookie sheet.

Per cookie of 2 dozen
  Exchanges: 0.5 Bread, 1.25 Fat; 108 Calories, 2 g protein (7%), 7 g fat (56%),
10.5 g carbohydrate (37%; 3 g sugars), 1 g dietary fiber, 10 mg cholesterol, 12 mg sodium, $.15

VARIATIONS

Replace fructose with **¼ cup honey.**
Replace almonds with **1 cup pecans or walnuts, finely chopped.**

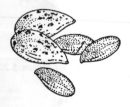

*Put some of the best products in your
bags and take them down to the man as
a gift--a little balm and a little honey,
some spices and myrrh, some pistachio
nuts and almonds. Genesis 43:11*

Apricot Dream Bars

A no-wheat, no sugar recipe and very rich! Cut into small "finger bars." I use Sorrel Ridge Fruit Spread for these, available at supermarkets, but any brand is suitable.

AMOUNT: 8" or 9" Square Bake Pan (36 Finger Bars)
Bake 300° for 45 minutes

1. Preheat oven to 300°.

2. Blend first cup oats and walnuts until fine in blender; combine evenly in mixing bowl with remaining oats, butter and cinnamon:
   1 cup *Quick Quaker Oats*, uncooked
   1 cup walnuts
   1 cup *Quick Quaker Oats*, uncooked
   1 stick (½ cup) butter, melted *(unsalted preferred, p. 32)*
   ½ teaspoon cinnamon

3. Press slightly more than half this mixture with a fork into 8" or 9" square pan for bottom layer; reserve remainder for the top.

4. Whisk together until smoothly blended; spread evenly over bottom layer with a spoon:
   8 oz. light cream cheese or cream cheese (stirred until soft)
   ½ cup skim milk ricotta cheese
   ½ teaspoon vanilla

5. Turn fruit spread into mixing bowl; stir vigorously to make easily spreadable; spread evenly over top of cream cheese mixture with a spoon (layer will be thin):
   10 oz. jar apricot all-fruit spread (or flavor desired) *(p. 41)*

6. Crumble **reserved crumb mixture** evenly over top of fruit spread with fingers (patiently!). Evenly distribute and press slightly down with a fork.

7. Bake in preheated oven at 300° for about 45 minutes. Cool thoroughly; refrigerate until cold before cutting into bars. Cut 9 x 4.

Per bar of 36
   Exchanges: 0.25 Meat, 0.25 Bread, 1.25 Fat, 0.25 Fruit; 97 Calories, 2.5 g protein (11%), 6.5 g fat (58%), 7.5 g carbohydrate (31%; 4 g sugars), 0.5 g dietary fiber, 12 mg cholesterol, 28 mg sodium, $.20

Date Sugar Cookies

A delicately crisp cookie, not too sweet. This will give you the experience of using date sugar, a good replacement for brown sugar; but use brown sugar if you do not have access to date sugar.

AMOUNT: About 2 Dozen
Bake 350° for 10-12 minutes

1. Whisk butter and sugar together until well mixed; whisk in egg, honey and vanilla:
   - **1 stick (½ cup) soft butter** *(unsalted preferred, p. 32)*
   - **½ cup date sugar, packed** *(p. 13)* **or brown sugar, packed**
   - **1 egg** *(or alternative, p. 39)*
   - **3 tablespoons honey**
   - **½ teaspoon vanilla**

2. Blend dry ingredients in separate bowl:
   - **1¾ cups whole wheat pastry flour** *(p. 14; or alternative, pp. 20-22)*
   - **1 teaspoon baking soda**

3. Blend dry ingredients into liquid ingredients. Chill dough for easier handling, if needed.

4. Roll tablespoons of dough into walnut-size balls with palms of hands or dispense with all-purpose scoop (p. 48); place on ungreased cookie sheet.

5. Bake in preheated oven at 350° for 10-12 minutes until almost no imprint remains when touched lightly. Remove immediately from cookie sheet.

Per cookie of 2 dozen
   Exchanges: 0.5 Bread, 0.75 Fat, 0.25 Fruit; 89 Calories, 1.5 g protein (6%), 4 g fat (41%), 12.5 g carohydrate (53%; 4 g sugars), 1.5 g dietary fiber, 19 mg cholesterol, 38 mg sodium, $.10

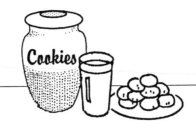

Candy No-Bake Cookies

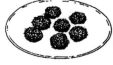

*I came across this one in the home of a friend, to whom I had given it 25 years ago but had forgotten! "This looks yummy," I said to myself, "with a few nutritional improvements, I can put it in **Desserts**." And so I did! Rich and yummy! Make it all in the same pan.*

AMOUNT: About 26 Cookies

1. In saucepan stir butter, *Sucanat* and dates together; don't worry that the *Sucanat* does not blend in well at this point:
   1 stick (½ cup) butter, melted *(unsalted preferred, p. 32)*
   ¾ cup *Sucanat* *(p. 14)*
   1 cup finely chopped date dices or nuggets *(p. 13)*
   (dice fine in the blender)

2. Heat and stir mixture constantly about 5 minutes until it follows the spoon around the pan; remove from heat and stir together until well blended.

3. Stir in and cook for 2 minutes:
   1 tablespoon milk *(or alternative, p. 39)*
   ½ teaspoon salt
   1 egg, well beaten *(or alternative, p. 39)*

4. Remove from heat and blend in thoroughly with mixing spoon:
   ½ teaspoon vanilla
   2 cups crispy brown rice cereal *(see Whole Grain Breakfast Cereals, p. 22)*
   ½ cup chopped walnuts

5. Cool mixture until easy to handle. Roll in walnut-size balls or use an all-purpose dispenser to scoop out portion for each ball (p. 55). Roll each ball until well coated in:
   1¼ cups medium shred or thread coconut, unsweetened *(p. 13)*

6. Place balls on a cookie sheet lined with wax paper; refrigerate. When well chilled, place in covered storage container or plastic bag and keep refrigerated.

Per cookie of 26
   Exchanges: 0.25 Bread, 1 Fat, 0.25 Fruit; 105 Calories, 1 g protein (6%), 6.5 g fat (52%), 12 g carbohydrate (43%; 8 g sugars), 1.5 g dietary fiber, 18 mg cholesterol, 48 mg sodium, $.15

VARIATION

Reduce butter to ½ **stick (¼ cup) butter** (less rich, but good). Replace *Sucanat* with ½ **cup honey.**

Per cookie of 26
   Exchanges: 0.25 Bread, 0.75 Fat, 0.25 Fruit; 85 Calories, 1 g protein (5%), 3.5 g fat (37%), 13 g carbohydrate (58%; 10 g sugars), 1.5 g dietary fiber, 11 mg cholesterol, 48 mg sodium, $.15

Carob or Chocolate Brownies

 So quick and easy to make. Mix everything in one saucepan except for mixing dry ingredients. For a lowfat cocoa powder option, see p. 42.

AMOUNT: 8" or 9" Square Pan (About 16 Bars)
Bake 325° for 40-45 minutes

1. Preheat oven to 325°. Grease or spray baking pan with non-stick spray (p. 54).

2. In saucepan whisk honey and butter until blended and creamy; whisk in eggs and vanilla:
   6 tablespoons melted butter *(unsalted preferred, p. 32)*
   ¾ cup honey
   2 eggs *(or alternative, p. 39)*
   1 teaspoon vanilla

3. Blend dry ingredients in small mixing bowl:
   1 cup whole wheat pastry flour *(p. 14; or alternative, pp. 20-22)*
   ½ cup cocoa or carob powder *(p. 13)*
      (stir through strainer to remove lumps)
   1½ teaspoons baking powder *(low sodium or Rumford preferred, p. 13)*
   1/8 teaspoon salt

4. Stir dry ingredients into liquid ingredients; stir in:
   ½ cup chopped walnuts, optional

5. Pour into baking pan. Bake in preheated oven at 325° for 40-45 minutes until knife comes out just clean (do not overbake).

Per brownie of 16 (pan cut 4 x 4), with cocoa powder, walnuts not included
   Exchanges: 0.25 Meat, 0.5 Bread, 1 Fat; 138 Calories, 2.5 g protein (7%), 5.5 g fat (34%)
21.5 g carbohydrate (59%; 13 g sugars), 1 g dietary fiber, 38 mg cholesterol, 28 mg sodium, $.20

Per brownie of 16 (pan cut 4 x 4), with carob powder, walnuts not included
   Exchanges: 0.25 Meat, 0.75 Bread, 1 Fat; 141 Calories, 2 g protein (5%), 5 g fat (31%),
24 g carbohydrate (64%; 13 g sugars), 1 g dietary fiber, 38 mg cholesterol, 28 mg sodium, $.15

Walnuts add per bar of 16:
   Exchanges: 0.5 Fat; 24 Calories, 2 g fat, $.05

VARIATION
May bake at 350° for 25-30 minutes, if desired.

Carob or Chocolate No-Bake Cookies

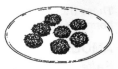

A very rich cookie. Fun for children to make. Make these either chocolate or carob, or half chocolate and half carob. Use less butter for lower fat or more for richer cookies.

AMOUNT: About 2 Dozen

1. Blend ingredients together in saucepan; heat over very low heat until butter melts; bring to boil and boil for 1 minute:
    ½ cup nonfat milk *(or alternative, p. 39)*
    ¼ - ½ cup butter *(unsalted preferred, p. 32)*
    2 - 1 oz. squares unsweetened chocolate
       or 1/3 cup carob powder *(p. 13)* **+ ¼ cup water**
       or 1 square chocolate + 3 Tbsps. carob + 2 Tbsps. water

2. Remove from heat and mix in, in order given:
    ½ cup honey
    1 teaspoon vanilla
    ¼ - ½ cup nonfat dry milk powder, optional *(p. 14)*
    3 cups *Quick* or *Old Fashioned* Quaker Oats *(see tip below)*

3. Drop by spoonfuls or dispense with all-purpose scoop (p. 48) onto cookie sheet lined with wax paper. Chill until firm in freezer or refrigerator. Keep refrigerated.

Per cookie of 2 dozen __with carob__   Exchanges: 0.5 Bread, 0.75 Fat; 97 Calories, 3 g protein (11%), 4 g fat (33%), 14.5 g carbohydrate (56%; 6 g sugars), 1 g dietary fiber, 6 mg cholesterol, 8 mg sodium, $.10

Per cookie of 2 dozen __with chocolate__   Exchanges: 0.75 Bread, 0.5 Fat; 91 Calories, 2.5 g protein (11%), 2.5 g fat (25%), 15.5 g carbohydrate (64%; 6 g sugars), 1 g dietary fiber, 6 mg cholesterol, 8 mg sodium, $.15

VARIATIONS

Add **½ cup peanut butter** *(p. 43)* before adding oats.
Add **½ cup chopped peanuts, walnuts, filberts, almonds, or sunflower seeds.**
Add **½-1 cup unsweetened coconut** *(p. 13)*.
For "health-packed" cookie use in place of ½ cup oats:
    ¼ cup toasted wheat germ *(p. 15)*
    3 tablespoons lecithin granules *(p. 14)*
    2 tablespoons brewer's yeast *(p. 13)*

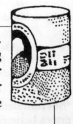

About Rolled Oats: *Quick* oats are finer than *Old Fashioned* oats. In most recipes they may be used interchangeably. Choose according to the texture you prefer. I list first what I prefer–*Quick* oats, for example, in the recipe above; my daughter Sharon, on the other hand, prefers *Old Fashioned* oats. *Quaker* is merely the brand name most commonly known. Any similar rolled oats will do.

Carob or Chocolate Chip Cookies

These thin, rich cookies are delicately crisp with Sucanat and softer with honey. Optional oats added makes a rounder, plumper cookie.

AMOUNT: About 34 Cookies (44 Cookies with Oats)
Bake 350° (375° with Oats) for 8-10 minutes

1. Preheat oven to 350° or 375°. Grease or spray cookie sheet (p. 54).

2. Whisk together until well blended and smooth:
   2/3 cup soft unsalted butter or ½ cup canola oil *(p. 13)*
   1 cup *Sucanat* *(p. 14)* **or ½ cup honey or crystalline fructose** *(p. 13)*

3. Whisk in:
   1 egg *(or alternative, p. 39)*
   1 teaspoon vanilla

4. Blend dry ingredients in separate bowl; stir into liquid ingredients:
   1¾ cups whole wheat pastry flour *(p. 14; or alternative, pp. 20-22)*
   ½ teaspoon baking soda
   ½ teaspoon salt

5. Stir in to blend well:
   1 cup *Quick Quaker Oats*, uncooked, optional *(see tip, p. 89)*
   ½ - 1 cup chocolate or carob chips *(p. 13)*
   ½ cup chopped walnuts, optional

6. Chill dough, if needed, for easy handling. Drop tablespoons of dough or dispense with all-purpose scoop (p. 48) onto cookie sheet leaving room between cookies to spread.

7. Bake in preheated oven at 350° (375° with oats) for 8-10 minutes. Cool 5 minutes before removing from cookie sheet. If made with oats immediately remove from sheet.

Per cookie of 44, with ½ cup chocolate chips, oats; without walnuts
  Exchanges: 0.5 Bread, 0.75 Fat; 76 Calories, 1 g protein (6%), 4 g fat (43%),
10 g carbohydrate (51%; 6 g sugars), 1 g dietary fiber, 12 mg cholesterol, 36 mg sodium, $.08*

Per cookie of 34, with ½ cup chocolate chips; without walnuts, oats
  Exchanges: 0.25 Bread, 1 Fat; 89 Calories, 1 g protein (5%), 5 g fat (46%),
11.5 g carbohydrate (49%; 6 g sugars), 0.5 g dietary fiber, 16 mg cholesterol, 47 mg sodium, $.09*

Per cookie of 34, with ½ cup carob chips; without walnuts, oats
  Exchanges: 0.5 Bread, 1 Fat; 89 Calories, 1 g protein (5%), 4.5 g fat (44%),
11.5 g carbohydrate (51%; 6 g sugars), 0.5 g dietary fiber, 16 mg cholesterol, 46 mg sodium, $.10

*Not rounded off upward to nearest $.05 in order to illustrate the difference in prices between this recipe and "fat free" recipes on p. 91.

"Fat-Free" Oatmeal Cookies

Adapted from recipe, p. 90, but fat-free--meaning no butter or oil has been added. This is just a sample of how you can alter many recipes to be fat free. These will have just a bit more of that "health food" taste, but we still really like them!   See pp. 32-33 for more information.

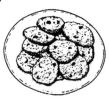

AMOUNT: About 40 Cookies
Bake 375° for 8-10 minutes

1. Preheat oven to 350°. Grease or spray cookie sheet (p. 54).

2. Whisk together until well blended and smooth:
   1 egg *(or alternative, p. 39)*
   ¼ cup water
   1 teaspoon vanilla
   1 cup Sucanat *(p. 14)*

3. Blend dry ingredients in separate bowl; stir into liquid ingredients:
   1¾ cups whole wheat pastry flour *(p. 14; or alternative, pp. 20-22)*
   ½ teaspoon baking soda
   ½ teaspoon salt

4. Stir in to blend well:
   ½ - 1 cup raisins or chocolate or carob chips *(p. 13)*
   1 cup Quick Quaker Oats, uncooked, optional *(see tip, p. 89)*

5. Chill dough, if needed, for easy handling. Drop tablespoons of dough or dispense with all-purpose scoop (p. 48) onto cookie sheet leaving room to spread.

6. Bake in preheated oven at 350° for 8-10 minutes. Cool 5 minutes before removing from cookie sheet.

Per cookie of 40, with ½ cup raisins; includes oats
  Exchanges: 0.5 Bread; 52 Calories, 1 g protein (9%), 0.5 g fat (7%),
  11.5 g carbohydrate (84%; 5 g sugars), 1 g dietary fiber, 5 mg cholesterol, 39 mg sodium, $.06*

VARIATION WITH LIQUID SWEETENER

Replace *Sucanat* with:
   1 cup Mystic Lake Dairy Mixed Fruit Concentrate Sweetener *(p. 28).*
Omit water.
Increase flour to **2¼ cups whole wheat pastry flour.**

Per cookie of 40, with ½ cup chocolate chips; includes oats
  Exchanges: 0.5 Bread, 0.25 Fat; 69 Calories, 1.5 g protein (8%), 1 g fat (16%)
  14 g carbohydrate (77%; 6 g sugars), 1 g dietary fiber, 14 mg cholesterol, 42 mg sodium, $.12*

*Not rounded off upward to nearest $.05 in order to illustrate the difference in prices between these recipes and recipe on p. 90.

Carob or Chocolate Drop Cookies

A very soft frosted cookie, not over-sweet , not too chocolaty. Nut piece on top especially makes easy to cover and store. If oil is used, dough is very soupy; refrigerating dough will make it easy to drop, though still soft. Cookies do not spread flat. For a lowfat cocoa powder option, see p. 42.

AMOUNT: About 3 Dozen
Bake 400° for 8-10 minutes

1. Whisk together oil or butter until thoroughly blended; whisk in remaining ingredients:
   ½ cup canola oil *(p. 13)* **or soft butter** *(unsalted preferred, p. 32)*
   ½ cup honey
   1 egg *(or alternative, p. 39)*
   1 teaspoon vanilla
   ¾ cup buttermilk *(or alternative, p. 39)*

2. Thoroughly blend in a separate bowl, stirring cocoa or carob through a strainer to remove any lumps:
   2 cups whole wheat pastry flour *(p. 14; or alternative, pp. 20-22)*
   6 tablespoons cocoa or carob powder *(p. 13)*
   ½ teaspoon baking soda
   ¼ teaspoon salt

3. Blend dry ingredients into liquid ingredients. Batter will be soupy, but can be immediately dropped on sheet with a all-purpose dispenser (p. 48); otherwise chill until easy to handle.

4. Preheat oven to 400°. Drop tablespoons of dough or dispense with all-purpose scoop onto greased cookie sheet. Bake 8-10 minutes. Remove cookies immediately from sheet; cool thoroughly before frosting.

5. **Frosting** Blend until smooth; spread over top of cooled cookies:
   1 stick (½ cup) soft butter *(unsalted preferred, p. 32)*
   5 Tbsps. (¼ cup with carob) crystalline fructose *(p. 13)*
   ¼ cup cocoa or carob powder (stir through strainer)
   1 teaspoon vanilla

6. Optional--Top each frosted cookie with **walnut piece or almond.**

Per cookie of 3 dozen with cocoa or carob, using 1% fat buttermilk and ½ walnut piece
Exchanges: 0.5 Bread, 1.25 Fat; 116 Calories, 2 g protein (6%), 6.5 g fat (51%),
13 g carbohydrate (43%; 6 g sugars), 1 g dietary fiber, 13 mg cholesterol, 35 mg sodium, $.15

VARIATIONS

~ Omit frosting; add **½ cup chopped walnuts or slivered almonds.**
~ Replace wheat flour with **Kamut flour** *(p. 13)*; chill cookies in refrigerator or freezer before eating for improved flavor.

Cinnamon Crisps

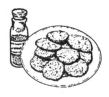

Delicately crisp. There is no leavening in these cookies so take extra care not to overmix. Baked cookies are especially flavorful if eaten chilled from the refrigrator.

AMOUNT: About 3 Dozen
Bake 350° for 10-12 minutes

1. Whisk together until well blended and creamy:
   1 stick (½ cup) soft butter *(unsalted preferred, p. 32)*
   ½ cup honey

2. Whisk in to mix evenly:
   ½ cup toasted wheat germ *(p. 15)*
   3 - 6 teaspoons cinnamon, to taste
   ½ teaspoon salt

3. Stir in:
   1½ cups whole wheat pastry flour *(p. 14; or alternative, pp. 20-22)*

4. Chill dough. Drop tablespoons of dough or dispense with all-purpose scoop (p. 48) onto ungreased cookie sheet, allowing plenty of room to spread.

5. Bake at 350° for 10-12 minutes. Cool 5 minutes before removing from cookie sheet.

Per cookie of 3 dozen   Exchanges: 0.5 Bread, 1 Fat; 86 Calories, 1 g protein (5%), 5.5 g fat (53%), 9.5 g carbohydrate (42%; 14 g sugars), 1 g dietary fiber, 14 mg cholesterol, 31 mg sodium, $.10

Peanut Clusters

AMOUNT: About 15 Pieces

1. Melt chocolate in saucepan over very low heat or in double boiler; remove from heat and blend in remaining ingredients:
   1 oz. square unsweetened chocolate
   1 teaspoon water
   3 tablespoons honey
   1 tablespoon *Sucanat* *(p. 14)* **or crystalline fructose** *(p. 13)*
   1/16 teaspoon salt
   1/8 teaspoon vanilla

2. Stir in to coat evenly:
   1 cup roasted, unsalted peanuts *(see toasted almonds tip, p. 13)*

3. Chill for 30 minutes for easier handling. Roll walnut-size pieces or dispense with all-purpose scoop (p. 48); set on wax paper; chill.

Per piece of 15
   Exchanges: 0.5 Bread, 1 Fat; 86 Calories, 1 g protein (5%), 5.5 g fat (53%), 9.5 g carbohydrate (42%; 4 g sugars), 1 g dietary fiber, 14 mg cholesterol, 31 mg sodium, $.15

Coconut Macaroons

Easy to make and so-o-o good! A macaroon is a cookie made of egg whites, sugar, usually almond paste or coconut, and sometimes a little flour (Random House Dictionary).

AMOUNT: About 2½ Dozen
Bake 325° for 20 minutes

1. Preheat oven to 325°. Lightly grease or spray cookie sheet (p. 54).

2. Mix together well with mixing spoon:
   2 2/3 cups (7 oz.) coconut, medium shred unsweetened *(p. 13)*
   ½ cup crystalline fructose *(p. 13)*
   ¼ cup whole wheat pastry flour *(p. 14; or alternative, pp. 20-22)*
      (or ¼ cup unbleached white flour)
   ¼ teaspoon salt

3. Whisk in thoroughly:
   4 egg whites, unbeaten
   1 teaspoon almond extract

4. Stir in, mixing well:
   1 cup finely chopped almonds *(p. 43)*

5. Drop tablespoons of dough or dispense with all-purpose scoop (p. 48) onto lightly greased cookie sheet; press together slightly with fingers (mixture will not hold together well until after baking).

6. Bake in preheated oven at 325° for 20 minutes or until just golden brown.

7. Immediately remove from cookie sheet to cool.

Per cookie of 2½ dozen
   Exchanges: 0.25 Meat, 0.25 Bread, 1 Fat; 84 Calories, 2 g protein (8%), 6 g fat (62%), 6.5 g carbohydrate (30%; 3 g sugars), 2 g dietary fiber, 0 mg cholesterol, 27 mg sodium, $.15

About Coconut: Coconut meat is a good source of dietary fiber, high quality protein, vitamine E, and minerals, including iron and iodine. Chewed well it is a good builder of muscle tissue, and provides energy. It is beneficial for several intestinal problems of the digestive tract such as constipation, gas, inflammation, and dysentery, and even assists in the destruction of worms, including tapeworm. Isn't that just like our God to have created these useful healing properties in such an important edible tropical fruit? His love endures forever!

Date Almond Granola Bars

AMOUNT: 9' x 13" Pan (2 Dozen Bars)
Bake 350° for 25-30 minutes

1. Preheat oven to 350°. Grease or spray pan (p. 54).

2. Whisk together until thoroughly blended:
   1 stick (½ cup) melted unsalted butter or ½ cup canola oil *(p. 13)*
   ½ cup honey

3. Toss together and blend into honey-butter mixture:
   4 cups *Quick Quaker Oats*, uncooked *(see tip, p. 89)*
   1 cup chopped almonds
   1 cup date dices or nuggets *(p. 13)* **or chopped dates** *(see tip, p. 71)*
   1 teaspoon cinnamon

4. Beat until stiff, but not dry, in electric mixer on high speed;
   fold into granola mixture:
   3 medium or 2 large egg whites
   (or 4 medium or 3 large whole eggs, beaten)

5. Press into greased pan and bake in preheated oven at 350°
   for 25-30 minutes.

6. Press down with rubber spatula; cool; cut into bars, 6 x 4.

Per bar of 2 dozen
   Exchanges: 0.25 Meat, 0.75 Bread, 1.25 Fat, 0.25 Fruit; 167 Calories, 4.5 g protein (10%),
   8 g fat (40%), 22 g carbohydrate (50%; 10 g sugars), 2 g dietary fiber, 10 mg cholesterol,
   8 mg sodium, $.20

Simple Granola Bars

AMOUNT: 8" or 9" Square Pan (1 Dozen Bars)
Bake 350° for 29-30 minutes

1. Preheat oven to 350°. Grease or spray pan (p. 54).

2. Blend remaining ingredients into beaten eggs:
   2 beaten eggs
   2 cups favorite granola or *Simple Granola* *(Breakfasts, p. 116)*
   ½ cup chopped nuts or dried fruit, optional

3. Press into greased pan and bake in preheated oven at 350°
   for 20-30 minutes.

4. Cool and cut into bars, 3 x 4.

Per bar of 1 dozen, with Simple Granola, does not include fruit or nuts
   Exchanges: 0.25 Meat, 0.75 Bread, 0.5 Fat; 98 Calories, 3.5 g protein (14%), 4 g fat (36%),
   12.5 g carbohydrate (50%; 3 g sugars), 1.5 g dietary fiber, 36 mg cholesterol, 12 mg sodium, $.10

Date Walnut Cookies

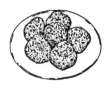

A wheatless cookie developed from the list of ingredients on a commercial brand. Not overly sweet. The coriander is an unusual flavor for a cookie, not pleasing to my taste until the cookies are refrigerator-cold and aged a day--after which they are very enjoyable.

AMOUNT: About 3½ Dozen
Bake 375° for 8-10 minutes

1. Preheat oven to 375°. Grease or spray cookie sheet (p. 54).

2. Whisk thoroughly to blend well:
    ½ cup soft unsalted butter or ½ cup canola oil *(p. 13)*
    1 cup *Sucanat* *(p. 14)* **or ½ cup crystalline fructose** *(p. 13)*
    2 eggs *(or alternative, p. 39)*
    1 teaspoon vanilla

3. In separate bowl blend dry ingredients; stir into liquid ingredients with mixing spoon to combine well:
    1 cup barley flour *(from whole hulled barley preferred, p. 13)*
    ½ cup brown rice flour *(p. 13)*
    ¼ cup oat bran
    1 teaspoon ground coriander
    1 teaspoon baking soda
    ½ teaspoon salt

4. Stir in until evenly mixed:
    1 cup *Quick Quaker Oats*, uncooked *(see tip, p. 89)*
    ½ cup date dices or nuggets *(p. 13)* **or chopped dates** *(see tip, p. 71)*
    ½ cup chopped walnuts

5. Drop tablespoons of dough or dispense with all-purpose scoop (p. 48) onto greased cookie sheet, leaving room for moderate spreading.

6. Press cookies lightly with floured fork to flatten a bit.

7. Bake in preheated oven at 375° for 8-10 minutes until golden brown. Remove immediately from cookie sheet to cool.

Per cookie of 3½ dozen
 Exchanges: 0.5 Bread, 0.5 Fat; 78 Calories, 1.5 g protein (9%), 3.5 g fat (40%),
10 g carbohydrate (51%; 5 g sugars), 1 g dietary fiber, 16 mg cholesterol, 49 mg sodium, $.10

VARIATION
    Replace barley flour, brown rice flour, and oat bran with:
    1¾ cups whole wheat pastry flour

Emilie's Yummy Oatmeals

Rich and delicious morsels that stand up in little mounds,
these contain the works!

AMOUNT: About 4 Dozen (5 Dozen with Coconut)
Bake 350° for 10-12 minutes

1. Preheat oven to 350°. Grease or spray cookie sheet (p. 54).

2. Whisk butter and honey together until well blended and creamy; whisk in egg:
    1 stick (½ cup) soft butter *(unsalted preferred, p. 32)*
    2/3 cup honey
    1 egg *(or alternative, p. 39)*

3. Blend dry ingredients in a separate bowl:
    1 cup whole wheat pastry flour *(p. 14; or alternative, pp. 20-22)*
    1 teaspoon cinnamon
    ½ teaspoon baking soda
    ½ teaspoon salt
    ¼ teaspoon nutmeg

4. With mixing spoon stir dry ingredients into liquid ingredients just until evenly mixed.

5. Stir in until evenly mixed:
    2 cups *Quick Quaker Oats*, uncooked *(see tip, p. 89)*
    1 cup raisins
    1 cup carob chips *(p. 13)* **or chocolate chips**
    1 cup date dices or nuggets *(p. 13)* **or chopped dates** *(see tip, p. 71)*
    1 cup chopped walnuts
    1 cup coconut, unsweetened, optional *(p. 13)*
      (macaroon or medium shred)

6. Drop tablespoons of dough or dispense with all-purpose scoop (p. 48) onto lightly greased cookie sheet close together (these do not spread). If dough does not hold together well, press each dropped cookie together a bit with finger tips after filling up the cookie sheet.

7. Bake in preheated oven at 350° for 10-12 minutes. Cool before removing from cookie sheets.

Per cookie of 4 dozen with carob chips; coconut excluded
    Exchanges: 0.5 Bread, 0.75 Fat, 0.25 Fruit; 108 Calories, 2 g protein (8%), 4.5 g fat (36%), 16 g carbohydrate (36%; 10 g sugars), 1.5 g dietary fiber, 5 mg cholesterol, 32 mg sodium, $.15

Per cookie of 5 dozen with chocolate chips; includes coconut
    Exchanges: 0.25 Bread, 0.75 Fat, 0.25 Fruit; 93 Calories, 1.5 g protein (7%), 4.5 g fat (42%), 13 g carbohydrate (52%; 9 g sugars), 1.5 g dietary fiber, 4 mg cholesterol, 26 mg sodium, $.10

Frosted Pumpkin Gems

These frosted cake-like cookies are perfectly special for a party!

AMOUNT: About 4 Dozen
Bake 350° for 15 minutes

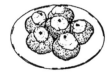

1. Preheat oven to 350°. Grease or spray cookie sheets with non-stick spray (p. 54).

2. Whisk together until well blended and creamy:
    1/3 cup soft butter *(unsalted preferred, p. 32)*
    2/3 cup honey, *Sucanat (p. 14)* **or crystalline fructose** *(p. 13)*

3. Whisk in thoroughly:
    2 eggs *(or alternative, p. 39)*
    1 cup canned pumpkin (8 oz. can or ½ -16 oz. can)
    ½ cup unsweetened applesauce
    2 teaspoons vanilla

4. Blend dry ingredients in separate bowl:
    3 cups whole wheat pastry flour *(p. 14; or alternative, pp. 20-22)*
    3 teaspoons cinnamon
    3 teaspoons allspice
    2 teaspoons baking powder *(low sodium or Rumford preferred, p. 13)*
    1 teaspoon baking soda
    ½ teaspoon salt

5. Whisk dry ingredients into liquid ingredients, blending well. Dough will be soft.

6. Drop tablespoons of dough or dispense with all-purpose scoop (p. 48) onto lightly greased cookie sheet, allowing at least an inch between (these spread a little).

7. Bake in preheated oven at 350° for 15 minutes until lightly browned. Remove cookies immediately from sheet to cool.

8. For **Cream Cheese Frosting** blend together thoroughly and spread 1½ teaspoons on each completely cooled cookie:
    8 oz. (1 cup) soft light cream cheese or cream cheese
    ½ stick (¼ cup) soft butter *(unsalted preferred, p. 32)*
    ¼ cup honey or crystalline fructose *(p. 13)*
    1 teaspoon orange extract

9. Optional--Top each cookie with **small piece pecan or walnut.**

Per cookie of 4 dozen, with about ½ piece of pecan half
    Exchanges: 0.5 Bread, 0.75 Fat; 94 Calories, 2 g protein (7%), 4 g fat (38%),
    13.5 g carbohydrate (55%; 6 g sugars), 1 g dietary fiber, 14 mg cholesterol, 63 mg sodium, $.15

Gingerbread People

A special holiday cookie. Children will especially enjoy making these! Choose the strength of molasses you prefer for flavor (see p. 27).

AMOUNT: Varies with Size of Cookie Cutters
Bake 350° for 10-12 minutes

1. Whisk together first 3 ingredients; beat in eggs to blend well:
   1 stick (½ cup) soft butter *(unsalted preferred, p. 32)*
   1 cup molasses *(p. 27)*
   2 tablespoons honey
   4 eggs

2. Blend dry ingredients in separate bowl; with mixing spoon blend well into liquid ingredients, but do not overmix:
   4 cups whole wheat pastry flour *(p. 14)*
   1½ teaspoons ground ginger
   1 teaspoon allspice
   1 teaspoon cinnamon
   ½ teaspoon nutmeg
   ½ teaspoon ground cloves
   3 teaspoons baking soda

3. Wrap dough in wax paper and chill for at least 1 hour.

4. Working with small amounts at a time, roll dough out 1/8"-¼" thick on a surface lightly dusted with flour, if needed, to prevent sticking. Cut dough with gingerbread people cookie cutters.

5. Place on lightly greased cookie sheets. Bake in preheated oven at 350° for 10-12 minutes. Remove immediately from cookie sheet to cool.

6. For **frosting** blend together thoroughly and frost completely cooled cookies:
   4 oz. soft light cream cheese, *Neufchatel,* or cream cheese
   ¼ cup plain nonfat yogurt
   1 tablespoon honey
   ½ teaspoon lemon juice
   ½ teaspoon vanilla

7. Decorate with **raisins** and **red hots**.

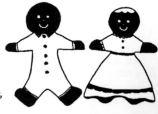

Per Recipe frosted, without raisins or red hots
   Exchanges: 4 Meat, 0.25 Milk, 28 Bread, 26.5 Fat;
4,339 Calories, 96.5 g protein (9%), 152.5 g fat (30%),
699 g carbohydrate (61%; 239 g sugars), 57.5 g dietary fiber,
1,189 mg cholesterol, 3,583 mg sodium, $5.00

Gingies

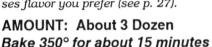

A firm chewy cookie with yummy spice flavor, these are best eaten fresh. If they become hard on standing, place in a paper bag with a few drops of water sprinkled inside, place in the oven for a few minutes at 300° and eat immediately. Choose the strength of molasses flavor you prefer (see p. 27).

AMOUNT: About 3 Dozen
Bake 350° for about 15 minutes

1. Whisk first 3 ingredients together thoroughly; whisk in water:
   3 tablespoons soft butter (*unsalted preferred, p. 32*)
   ¼ cup honey
   ¾ cup molasses (*p. 27*)
   1/3 cup cold water

2. Blend dry ingredients in separate bowl and blend into liquid ingredients:
   3¼ cups whole wheat pastry flour (*p. 14; or alternative, pp. 20-22*)
   ½ teaspoon allspice
   ½ teaspoon ground ginger
   ½ teaspoon ground cloves
   ½ teaspoon cinnamon
   1 teaspoon baking soda
   ½ teaspoon salt

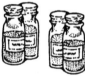

3. If you do not have a scoop dispenser, chill dough thoroughly for easy handling.

4. Preheat oven to 350°.

5. Roll tablespoons of dough in palms of hands or dispense with all-purpose scoop (p. 48), placing on lightly greased cookie sheet.

6. Press cookies out slightly with lighly floured fork.

7. Bake about 15 minutes. Remove immediately from cookie sheet to cool.

Per cookie of 3 dozen
*Exchanges: 0.75 Bread, 0.25 Fat; 75 Calories, 1 g protein (6%), 1 g fat (14%),
16 g carbohydrate (80%; 6 g sugars), 1.5 g dietary fiber, 3 mg cholesterol, 60 mg sodium, $.10*

Hobo Fortune Cookies

These thin dark cookies have a delightfully pleasant chewy texture. I like to store these in the freezer, removing them just a few minutes before serving. Choose the flavor strength of molasses you prefer (see p. 27). We like these with the strong flavor of blackstrap molasses.

AMOUNT: About 3 Dozen
Bake 375° for 8-9 minutes

1. Preheat oven to 375°. Grease or spray cookie sheet (p. 54).

2. Whisk the butter until very smooth and soft; whisk in sugar to blend well:
    ½ cup (1 stick) very soft butter *(unsalted preferred, p. 32)*
    1 cup *Sucanat (p. 14)* **or lightly packed brown sugar**

3. In liquid measuring cup stir baking soda into molasses:
    ¼ cup molasses *(unsulfured preferred, p. 27)*
    2 teaspoons baking soda

4. Whisk molasses into butter-sugar; whisk in to blend thoroughly:
    1 egg *(or alternative, p. 39)*

5. Blend dry ingredients in separate bowl; stir into liquid ingredients with mixing spoon until well blended:
    1½ cups whole wheat pastry flour *(p. 14; or alternative, pp. 20-22)*
    1½ teaspoons cinnamon
    ½ teaspoon ground cloves
    ¼ teaspoon ground ginger

6. Stir in, blending evenly:
    1 cup *Quick Quaker Oats*, **uncooked** *(see tip, p. 89)*

7. Drop tablespoons of dough or dispense with all-purpose scoop (p. 48) onto greased or sprayed cookie sheet, leaving plenty of room for spreading. These usually spread quite a bit.

8. Bake in preheated oven at 375° for 8-9 minutes. Allow to cool for 2-3 minutes before removing from cookie sheet.

Per cookie of 3 dozen
  Exchanges: 0.5 Bread, 0.5 Fat; 75 Calories, 1 g protein (6%), 3 g fat (34%), 11.5 g carbohydrate (60%; 5 g sugars), 1 g dietary fiber, 13 mg cholesterol, 51 mg sodium, $.10

> *. . . the kingdom of God is not a matter of eating and drinking, but of righteousness, peace and joy in the Holy Spirit.*
> Romans 14:17

Kamut-Oatmeal Cookies

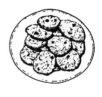

Satisfy your sweet tooth with this healthy yummy cookie with a very satisfying chewy texture! I prefer to use Sucanat (p. 14) for these.

AMOUNT: About 2½ Dozen
Bake 375° for 12 minutes

1. Cover raisins with water to soften; set aside:
   ½ cup raisins

2. Whisk together to blend thoroughly:
   ½ cup canola oil *(p. 13)* **or very soft unsalted butter**
   1 cup *Sucanat* *(p. 14)*
   1 egg *(or alternative, p. 39)*
   1½ teaspoons vanilla

3. Blend dry ingredients in separate bowl; mix into liquid ingredients:
   2/3 cup Kamut flour *(p 13)* **or whole wheat pastry flour** *(p. 14)*
   1 cup finely ground rolled oats
      (about 1 1/3 cups rolled oats ground in blender)
   ½ teaspoon baking powder *(low sodium or Rumford preferred, p. 13)*
   ½ teaspoon baking soda
   ¼ teaspoon salt

4. Stir oats into batter; fold in raisins and optional ingredients as desired:
   1 cup *Old Fashioned Quaker Oats*, uncooked *(see tip, p. 89)*
   ½ cup softened raisins, drained
   ½ cup chocolate or carob chips, optional *(p. 13)*
   ½ cup chopped walnuts, optional

5. Drop tablespoons of dough or dispense with all-purpose scoop onto greased cookie sheet allowing a couple inches between each cookie. Bake in preheated oven at 375° for about 12 minutes.

6. Immediately remove from cookie sheet to cool.

Per cookie of 2½ dozen with canola oil ; optional ingredients not included
   Exchanges: 0.5 Bread, 0.75 Fat; 94 Calories, 2 g protein (8%), 4.5 g. fat (40%),
13 g carbohydrate (52%; 7 g sugars), 1 g dietary fiber, 7 mg cholesterol, 34 mg sodium, $.10

Kamut Flake Cookies

These are quite sweet. Purchase the cereal at a health food store. There are other brands of Kamut flakes but I like Arrowhead Mills best.

   Replace oats in step #4 with **1-2 cups *Arrowhead Mills* Kamut Whole Grain Cereal** (flakes). Omit chips and nuts.

Mother's Little Secret Candies

High protein goodie! Note the high fiber content, too!
Fun for children to make. For a lowfat cocoa powder
option, see p.42.

AMOUNT: About 4 Dozen

1. Grind in blender, not more than 1 cup at a time
   (a coffee bean grinder is ideal for the seeds if you have one):
   3 cups roasted peanuts *(see tip for toasted almonds, p. 73)*
   ¾ cup sunflower seeds *(p. 14)*
   1/3 cup sesame seeds *(p. 14)*
   1/3 cup flax seeds *(p. 13)*

2. In mixing bowl whisk butter and honey together until well
   blended and creamy; blend in protein powder:
   1 stick (½ cup) soft butter *(unsalted preferred, p. 32)*
   1 cup honey
   1 cup protein powder *(tip, p. 111)* **or non-instant nonfat dry**
   milk powder *(p. 14)*

3. Evenly mix in ground nuts and seeds with mixing spoon.

4. Divide mixture in half.

5. Add to half the dough:
   2 - 6 teaspoons cinnamon, to taste
   1 - 3 teaspoons nutmeg, to taste

6. Add to other half, stirring powder through
   a strainer to remove lumps:
   carob *(p. 13)* **or cocoa powder, to taste**
   ¼ - ½ teaspoon vanilla, to taste

7. Mold candy pieces into a variety of shapes.

8. Store in freezer until shortly before serving.

Per candy of 24 <u>with 2 tsp. cinnamon, 1 tsp. nutmeg</u>
   Exchanges: 0.5 Meat, 0.25 Bread, 1.5 Fat; 121 Calories, 5 g protein (15%), 8.5 g fat (58%),
9 g carbohydrate (27%; 6 g sugars), 7.5 g dietary fiber, 5 mg cholesterol, 9 mg sodium, $.20

Per candy of 24 <u>with ½ tsp. vanilla, ¼ cup carob powder</u>
   Exchanges: 0.5 Meat, 0.25 Bread, 1.5 Fat; 125 Calories, 5 g protein (15%), 8.5 g fat (56%),
10 g carbohydrate (29%; 6 g sugars), 7.5 g dietary fiber, 5 mg cholesterol, 9 mg sodium, $.20

VARIATIONS

Experiment with other flavorings such as **mint, orange,**
   or almond extract, to taste in place of spices or vanilla or with
   coconut in place of carob or cocoa powder.

103

Nutty Millet Bars

A tasty "Rice Crispie Bar" alternative. Bags of puffed cold cereals are available in health food stores and in some supermarkets.

AMOUNT: 8" or 9" Square Pan (16 Bars)

1. Blend in blender until nuts and dates are tiny pieces; pour into mixing bowl:

   ¼ cup roasted unsalted peanuts *(see toasted almonds tip, p. 73)*
   ¼ cup almonds
   ¼ cup walnuts
   ¼ cup date dices or nuggets *(p. 13)* **or chopped dates** *(see tip, p. 71)*
   1½ teaspoons cinnamon

2. Grind peanuts in blender until blender will no longer grind efficiently; add remaining ingredients and blend until smooth:

   ½ cup roasted unsalted peanuts
   ½ stick (¼ cup) soft butter *(unsalted preferred, p. 32)*
   ½ cup honey
   1½ teaspoons vanilla

3. Blend butter-honey mixture into ground nut-date mixture. Stir in thoroughly:

   2½ cups puffed millet *(p. 13)*

4. Pat into 8" or 9" square baking pan; cover with wax paper. Chill thoroughly. Cut into bars, 4 x 4.

Per bar of 16
   Exchanges: 0.25 Meat, 0.25 Bread, 1.5 Fat, 0.25 Fruit; 137 Calories, 3 g protein (9%), 8.5 g fat (52%), 14.5 g carbohydrate (40%; 10 g sugars), 6 g dietary fiber, 8 mg cholesterol, 2 mg sodium, $.20

Carob Date Fudge

AMOUNT: About 3 Dozen Pieces

1. Whisk first 3 ingredients together thoroughly; gradually mix in remaining ingredients, one at a time, with mixing spoon; press into pan; chill; shape into balls or cut in squares:

   ½ stick (¼ cup) soft butter *(unsalted preferred, p. 32)*
   ½ cup honey
   3 teaspoons vanilla
   2/3 cup non-instant nonfat dry milk powder *(p. 14)*
   1/3 cup carob powder *(p. 13)* (stir through strainer to remove lumps)
   ½ cup date dices or nuggets *(p. 13)* **or dates, chopped small** *(p. 71)*
   ½ cup chopped walnuts

2. Optional--Roll balls in coconut or sesame seeds.

Per piece of 3 dozen without coconut or sesame seeds
   Exchanges: 0.5 Fat; 55 Calories, 1.5 g protein (10%), 2 g fat (35%), 8 g carbohydrate (55%; 6 g sugars), 0.5 g dietary fiber, 4 mg cholesterol, 13 mg sodium, $.10

Oatmeal Raisin Cookies

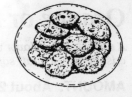

These little mounded morsels are delicately crisp made with Sucanat, but soft made with honey.

AMOUNT: About 3 Dozen
Bake 375° for 8-10 minutes

1. Cover raisins with water to soften:
   ½ cup raisins

2. Preheat oven to 375°. Grease or spray cookie sheet with non-stick spray (p. 54).

3. Whisk together until evenly mixed (with *Sucanat* this will still be crumbly; with honey it should be creamy):
   ½ stick (¼ cup) soft butter *(unsalted preferred, p. 32)*
   1 cup *Sucanat* *(p. 14)* **or ½ cup honey**

4. Whisk in, blending well:
   1 egg *(or alternative, p. 39)*
   1 teaspoon vanilla

5. Blend dry ingredients in a separate bowl; stir into liquid ingredients until well mixed:
   1 cup whole wheat pastry flour *(p. 14; or alternative, pp. 20-22)*
   ¼ cup soy, millet, or oat flour *(p. 13)*
   or additional ¼ cup pastry wheat or spelt flour *(p. 21)*
   1 teaspoon cinnamon
   1 teaspoon baking soda
   ½ teaspoon salt

6. Stir in (with *Sucanat* dough is quite stiff; to mix in oats, use a cutting motion with spoon through the dough to assist mixing):
   drained raisins
   2 cups *Old Fashioned Quaker Oats*, uncooked *(see tip, p. 89)*

7. Drop tablespoons of dough or dispense with all-purpose scoop (p. 48) onto greased cookie sheet. Dough made with *Sucanat* will be especially dry. I press the dough together as I scoop the mounds onto the sheet, assisting a little with my fingers. These usually don't spread much, so can be fairly close together.

8. Bake at 375° for 8-10 minutes until just firm and lightly browned. Remove immediately from cookie sheet to cool.

Per cookie of 3 dozen with ¼ cup soy flour
  Exchanges: 0.5 Bread, 0.25 fat; 71 Calories, 2 g protein (10%), 2 g fat (24%),
12 g carbohydrate (67%; 6 g sugars), 1 g dietary fiber, 9 mg cholesterol, 55 mg sodium, $.10

Orange or Lemon Spice Cookies

A delicate spice flavor with a hint of orange or lemon, these cookies will be crisp with Sucanat, soft with honey. My favorite cookie!

AMOUNT: About 2½ Dozen
Bake 375° for 8-10 minutes

1. Preheat oven to 375°. Grease or spray cookie sheet (p. 54).

2. Whisk together until thoroughly blended:
   1 stick (½ cup) very soft butter *(unsalted preferred, p. 32)*
   1 cup Sucanat *(p. 14)* **or ½ cup honey**

3. Whisk in until well blended:
   1 egg *(or alternative, p. 39)*
   1 teaspoon vanilla

4. Blend dry ingredients in separate bowl;
   stir into liquid ingredients (dough will be quite stiff with *Sucanat*):
   2 cups whole wheat pastry flour *(p. 14; or alternative, pp. 20-22)*
   1 tablespoon non-instant nonfat dry milk powder *(p. 14)*
   1 tablespoon grated lemon or orange peel *(see tip below)*
   ½ teaspoon cinnamon
   ½ teaspoon nutmeg
   1 teaspoon baking powder *(low sodium or Rumford preferred, p. 13)*
   ½ teaspoon baking soda

5. Chill dough if needed for easy handling. Drop tablespoons of dough or dispense with all-purpose scoop (p. 48) onto greased cookie sheet; leave at least 2 inches between cookies.

6 Flatten shaped dough slightly on cookie sheet with floured fork.

7. Sprinkle each cookie with **cinnamon sugar, optional** *(p. 115)* and top with **almond.**

8. Bake in preheated oven at 375° for 8-10 minutes until lightly browned.

9. Cool 2 minutes before removing from cookie sheet.

Per cookie of 2½ dozen, with 1/8 tsp. cinnamon sugar and almond
   Exchanges: 0.5 Bread, 0.75 Fat; 92 Calories, 1.5 g protein (6%), 4 g fat (38%),
13.5 g carbohydrate (56%; 5 g sugars), 1 g dietary fiber, 15 mg cholesterol, 18 mg sodium, $.15

Lemon/Orange Peel Storage Tip: Keep a small container of grated fresh lemon peel and/or orange peel in the freezer for ready use. This way you won't need to buy the fresh fruit just to have peel nor will you need to rely on the commercially available jars of dried peel that are less tasty and flavorful (especially after several months of storage in a cupboard).

Peanut Butter Sesame Cookies

Sesame seeds add a bit of nice crunch to this kid-pleasing peanut butter cookie. Made with Sucanat, they will be crisp, with honey, soft.

AMOUNT: About 3½ Dozen
Bake 350° for 12 minutes

1. Preheat oven to 350°. Grease or spray cookie sheet with non-stick spray (p. 54).

2. Whisk together until well blended and smooth:
   1 stick (½ cup) soft unsalted butter or ½ cup canola oil *(p. 13)*
   1 cup *Sucanat* *(p. 14)* **or ½ cup honey**
   1 egg *(or alternative, p. 39)*
   1 teaspoon vanilla
   2 tablespoons water
   1/3 cup sesame seeds *(p. 14)*
   ½ cup peanut butter *(p. 43)*

3. Blend dry ingredients in separate bowl:
   1½ cups whole wheat pastry flour *(p. 14; or alternative, pp. 20-22)*
   ½ cup non-instant nonfat dry milk powder *(p. 14)*
   1 teaspoon salt
   ½ teaspoon baking powder *(low sodium or Rumford preferred, p. 13)*

4. Stir dry ingredients into liquid ingredients until well blended. Dough with *Sucanat* will be quite stiff.

5. Stir in evenly:
   1 cup *Quick Quaker Oats*, **uncooked, optional** *(see tip, p. 89)*

6. If you don't have an all-purpose scoop (p. 48), chill dough made with honey until easy to roll in palms of hands without sticking.

7. Roll tablespoons of dough or dispense with all-purpose scoop onto lightly greased cookie sheet and flatten with floured fork (cookies will not usually spread much during baking).

8. Bake in preheated oven at 350° for about 12 minutes. Remove immediately from cookie sheet to cool.

Per cookie of 3½ dozen, includes oats
Exchanges: 0.25 Meat, 0.5 Bread, 0.75 Fat; 89 Calories, 2.5 g protein (11%), 4.5 g fat (44%), 10 g carbohydrate (44%; 4 g sugars), 1 g dietary fiber, 11 mg cholesterol, 80 mg sodium, $.10

VARIATION

Omit sesame seeds from dough; roll balls in sesame seeds before flattening with a fork on cookie sheet.

Persimmon Cookies

This glowing orange fruit ripens in time for Thanksgiving and Christmas seasons. I use the Hachiya variety grown mostly in California. These persimmons, about the size of a peach and slightly acorn-shaped, are ripe when very soft in contrast to the more squat Fuju or Japanese persimmon that may be eaten while still firm. The pulp freezes well for year-round use (see **Lunches & Snacks**, p. 69, for special tip on freezing). Cookies are spicy. One of my favorite cookies, these taste best chilled.

AMOUNT: About 4 Dozen
Bake 375° for 12-15 minutes

1. Preheat oven to 375°. Grease or spray cookie sheets with non-stick spray (p. 54).

2. Stir soda into persimmon pulp; set aside:
   1 cup ripe persimmon pulp (about 3 peeled persimmons)
   1 teaspoon baking soda

3. Whisk butter and honey together until well blended and creamy; whisk in eggs:
   1 stick (½ cup) soft butter (unsalted preferred, p. 32)
   ½ cup honey
   2 eggs (or alternative, p. 39)

4. Blend dry ingredients in separate bowl:
   2 cups whole wheat pastry flour (p. 14; or alternative, pp. 20-22)
   1 teaspoon cinnamon
   1 teaspoon ground cloves
   1 teaspoon nutmeg
   1 teaspoon baking powder (low sodium or Rumford preferred, p. 13)
   ½ teaspoon salt

5. Whisk persimmon pulp into liquid ingredients. Stir in dry ingredients just until thoroughly mixed; stir in evenly:
   1 cup chopped walnuts
   1 cup raisins

6. Dough will be quite soft. Drop tablespoons of dough or dispense with all-purpose scoop (p. 48) onto lightly greased cookie sheet leaving room between to spread.

7. Bake in preheated oven at 375° for 12-15 minutes. Immediately remove from cookie sheet to cool.

Per cookie of 4 dozen
Exchanges: 0.25 Bread, 0.75 Fat, 0.25 Fruit; 82 Calories, 1.5 g protein (7%), 4 g. fat (39%), 12 g carbohydrate (54%; 6 g sugars), 1 g dietary fiber, 14 mg cholesterol, 43 mg sodium, $.10

Polynesian Squares

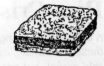

The reduced fat variation of this recipe, below, is the original. I thought it tasted a bit like health food so I increased the nuts, added some fat, and used wheat germ in place of flour. Both recipes passed the taste test of our small fellowship group. My changes had a slight edge in popularity, but several liked the original recipe just as well. They all thought these had apples in them. So call them Mock-Apple Squares if you like!

AMOUNT: 9" x 13" Pan (24 Squares)
Bake 350° for 30 minutes

1. Preheat oven to 350°.

2. Combine in saucepan; cook over low heat, stirring frequently until thickened and saucy, about 10-15 minutes:
   20 oz. can crushed unsweetened pineapple, drained
   2 cups date dices or nuggets (p. 13) **or chopped dates** (p. 71)
   3/8 cup (6 Tbsps.) drained pineapple juice

3. Thoroughly blend together in mixing bowl:
   3 cups *Quick Quaker Oats*, uncooked
   1 cup toasted wheat germ (p. 15)
   1 cup medium shred coconut, unsweetened (p. 13)
   1 cup chopped walnuts
   ¾ teaspoon salt
   1¼ cups juice (remaining drained pineapple juice + orange juice as needed, or more pineapple juice)
   ½ stick (¼ cup) butter, melted (*unsalted preferred, p. 32*)

4. Press half the dry mixture evenly in bottom of baking pan. Spread cooked sauce evenly over the top. Top with remaining dry mixture, pressing it down evenly over top of sauce.

5. Bake in preheated oven at 350° for 30 minutes or until lightly golden brown. Refrigerate until cold. Cut into squares.

Per square of 24
   Exchanges: 0.25 Meat, 1 Bread, 1.25 Fat, 1 Fruit; 185 Calories, 6 g protein (12%), 8 g fat (36%), 26 g carbohydrate (52%; 13 g sugars), 4 g dietary fiber, 5 mg cholesterol, 71 mg sodium, $.30

REDUCED FAT VARIATION

Omit butter. Reduce walnuts to **½ cup chopped walnuts**. Replace wheat germ with **1 cup millet flour or other whole grain flour** (p. 13).

Per square of 24 with millet flour
   Exchanges: 1 Bread, 0.5 Fat, 1 Fruit; 154 Calories, 4 g protein (10%), 4 g fat (23%), 28 g carbohydrate (68%; 13 g sugars), 3.5 g dietary fiber, 71 mg sodium, $.20

Rice Crispy Oat Cookies

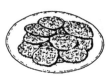

A delightfully crispy-chewy cookie and quite sweet. For these I use Grainfield's Whole Grain Crispy Brown Rice (a cold cereal, but not puffed) from the health food store.

AMOUNT: About 40
Bake 325° for 12-13 minutes

1. Whisk together until well blended and creamy, using the higher amount of butter for richer cookies:

   ½ - 1 stick (¼ -½ cup) soft butter (*unsalted preferred, p. 32*)
   ½ cup *Sucanat* (*p. 14*)
   1/3 cup crystalline fructose (*p. 13*)

2. Whisk in until well blended:

   1 egg (*or alternative, p. 39*)
   1 teaspoon vanilla

3. Blend dry ingredients in a separate bowl; mix into liquid ingredients:

   ¾ cup whole wheat pastry flour (*p. 14; or alternative, pp. 20-22*)
   ½ teaspoon baking powder (*low sodium or Rumford preferred, p. 13*)
   ½ teaspoon baking soda
   ¼ teaspoon salt

4. Stir in until evenly mixed:

   1¼ cups whole crispy brown rice cereal (*p. 22*)
   1 cup *Quick Quaker Oats*, uncooked (*see tip, p. 89*)
   ½ cup medium shred coconut, unsweetened (*p. 13*)

5. Dough may be chilled an hour, if desired.

6. Drop tablespoons of dough or dispense with all-purpose scoop (p. 48) onto greased cookie sheet leaving at least 2" between (these usually spread quite a bit).

7. Bake in preheated oven at 325° for 12-13 minutes. Allow to cool on cookie sheet 2-3 minutes for easier removal. These will be somewhat sticky, so be patient in removing them from the sheet.

8. Optional--For extra crispiness freeze the cookies before eating.

Per cookie of 40 <u>with ¼ cup butter</u>
  Exchanges: 0.25 Bread, 0.25 Fat; 52 Calories, 1 g protein (7%), 2 g fat (33%),
8 g carbohydrate (59%; 3 g sugars), 0.5 g dietary fiber, 8 mg cholesterol, 27 mg sodium, $.05

Per cookie of 40 <u>with ½ cup butter</u>
  Exchanges: 0.25 Bread, 0.5 Fat; 62 Calories, 1 g protein (6%), 3 g fat (44%),
8 g carbohydrate (50%; 3 g sugars), 0.5 g dietary fiber, 12 mg cholesterol, 27 mg sodium, $.10

Snowballs

A nutritious sweet morsel not to be heavily indulged in! Keep these chilled in the refrigerator or freezer until ready to serve. Purchase all ingredients at health food store except cream cheese and extract.

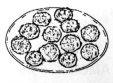

AMOUNT: About 4 Dozen Balls

1. Cover with boiling water; let stand 5 minutes to soften:
   1 cup dried apples

2. Soften cream cheese in electric mixer; blend in remaining ingredients:
   8 oz. light or *Neufchatel* cream cheese, cream cheese
   1¼ cups honey or crystalline fructose
   1½ cups non-instant nonfat dry milk powder
   ½ cup protein powder, optional *(see tip below)*
   or nonfat dry milk powder
   1 cup almonds, ground in blender
   1 cup sunflower seeds
   ½ cup macaroon coconut, unsweetened
   1 teaspoon almond extract
   softened dried apples, drained/chopped *(see tip, p. 71)*

3. Pat into 9" x 13" pan; freeze until very cold.

4. Cut into 48 small squares (6 x 8).

5. Roll each square into ball; roll in:
   macaroon coconut, unsweetened

6. Return to freezer or refrigerator until ready to serve.

Per ball of 4 dozen, coated with 1 tsp. coconut, <u>protein powder not included</u>
   Exchanges: 0.25 Meat, 0.25 Milk, 1 Fat; 110 Calories, 3.5 g protein (13%), 5.5 g fat (42%), 13 g carbohydrate (45%; 11 g sugars), 1 g dietary fiber, 13 mg cholesterol, 47 mg sodium, $.20

Per ball of 4 dozen, coated with 1 tsp. coconut, <u>with protein powder</u>
   Exchanges: 0.25 Meat, 0.25 Milk, 1 Fat; 108 Calories, 4 g protein (14%), 5.5 g fat (43%), 12 g carbohydrate (43%; 11 g sugars), 1 g dietary fiber, 4 mg cholesterol, 44 mg sodium, $.20

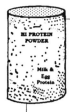

Protein Powder A high protein food supplement usually made from soy or milk-egg protein. I prefer the flavor of the latter. Most health food stores carry several brands with a wide range of flavor. If you live in southern California, I recommend *Trader Joe's Hi Protein Powder* for good flavor, available at Trader Joe Markets.

111

Tofu Spice Cookies

You will like these even if you don't like tofu.

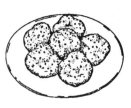

AMOUNT: About 4 Dozen
Bake 350° for 10-15 minutes

1. Place tofu between double layer of paper towel
   on a dinner plate to drain at least 30 minutes:
   14 oz. block tofu *(pp. 14, 15)*

2. Preheat oven to 350°. Grease or spray cookie sheet (p. 54).

3. Whisk butter and honey together until well blended
   and creamy; whisk in eggs and vanilla:
   1½ sticks (¾ cup) soft butter *(unsalted preferred, p. 32)*
   ¾ cup honey
   2 large eggs *(or alternative, p. 39)*
   2½ teaspoons vanilla

4. Crumble drained tofu with a fork and stir into liquid ingredients.

5. Blend dry ingredients in separate bowl:
   2 5/8 cups (2¼ c. + 2 Tbsp.) whole wheat pastry flour
   (p. 14; or alternative, pp. 20-22)
   2½ teaspoons ground ginger
   2½ teaspoons cinnamon
   1 teaspoon baking soda
   ¾ teaspoon salt

6. Blend dry ingredients into liquid
   ingredients just until mixed. Stir in evenly:
   ¾ cup raisins
   ¾ cup chopped walnuts
   ¾ cup date dices or nuggets *(p. 13)* **or chopped dates** *(see tip, p. 71)*

7. Drop tablespoons of dough or dispense with all-purpose scoop
   (p. 48) onto lightly greased cookie sheet (these usually do not
   spread much).

8. Bake in preheated oven at 350° for 10-15 minutes.
   Remove immediately from cookie sheet to cool.

Per cookie of 3 dozen
   Exchanges: 0.5 Bread, 0.75 Fat, 0.25 Fruit; 103 Calories, 2 g protein (8%), 4.5 g fat (37%)
15 g carbohydrate (54%; 8 g sugars), 1 g dietary fiber, 16 mg cholesterol, 55 mg sodium, $.15

Pies

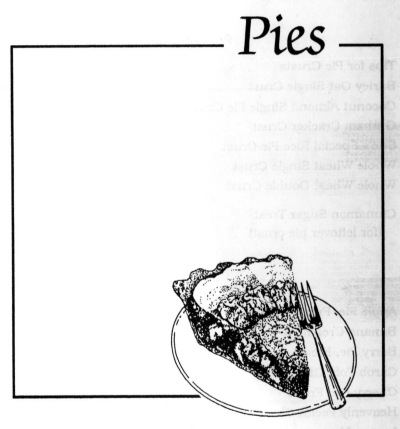

*By wisdom a house is built, and through understanding
it is established; through knowledge its rooms are filled
with rare and beautiful treasures
(Proverbs 24:3-4).
Rare and beautiful are the treasures
of nutrient-rich desserts!*

Pies

Mixing, Rolling, Shaping Pie Crust

These tips will help to produce successful flaky pie crusts.

MIXING

1. Whole wheat bread flour (not pastry, see p. 19) makes a more flaky and stable crust than pastry flour, but the latter also makes a good crust.
2. For a flaky crust, do not omit the salt.
3. Use almost refrigerator-cold butter, cut in ¼-½" pieces to assist mixing.
4. Cut the butter into the flour until the size of large peas, using pastry blender (p. 49) with twisting motion of the wrist.
5. Have water ice-cold. Add an ice cube for speedy chilling.
6. Mix water in with a fork, just until evenly mixed. Do not overmix. Dough will still be crumbly.
7. Gather dough together with hands, shaping into a ball in palms of hands, but handling as little as possible.

ROLLING

1. Slightly flatten ball of dough with palm of hand on piece of wax paper on counter top.
2. Cover with second piece wax paper and roll out with rolling pin from center outward.
3. While rolling, frequently flip the dough over to peel off paper on either side, replacing it each time; this will remove wrinkles in the paper and keep crust from sticking to it excessively. Gently pull paper close to the surface (if paper is lifted straight up, the crust is easily torn).
4. Form as even a circle as possible, large enough to fit bottom and sides of pie pan with a little over-hang on edges.
5. To place crust in the pie pan:
    a. Loosen top wax paper and replace it; flip crust over.
    b. Remove wax paper now on top. Crust still has paper underneath it.
    c. Lay the rolling pin on top of crust at one side; carefully, with a light hand, roll the crust onto the rolling pin while peeling away the wax paper.
    d. Set pie pan next to rolling pin; gently unroll crust from pin over top of plate. Don't worry if the crust cracks in a few places. This often happens with whole grain crust, especially when oil is used in the recipe.
6. Do not reroll dough as this toughens the texture.

SHAPING

1. Ease crust into pan so it is not stretched on the sides. Patch places where crust has cracked and add excess dough to places where crust does not quite reach a bit over edge of plate.
2. Trim around edges a little beyond plate edge with scissors or sharp knife.
3. Turn under edges, pinching dough to make a smooth rolled edge.
    Flute edge: For right-handed people--with left hand to left of pan edge, place forefinger and thumb on edge of crust; with right hand over the plate, extend forefinger between and pull dough toward the center; continue around entire edge of pan.
4. Prepare *Cinnamon-Sugar Treat* (p. 117), if desired, with leftover crust pieces.

Whole Wheat Single Pie Crust

We especially enjoy this crust with the wheat germ, although when rolled out it is a little more "breakable" than with all whole wheat. I prefer lightly salted butter for this to unsalted butter or oil. Butter gives better flavor and an easier-to-handle rolled out crust. See p. 115 for tips.

AMOUNT: 9½" Pie (for 9" Pie see tip below)
Bake 425° for 15-20 minutes *(prebaked crust only)*

1. Preheat oven to 425° if pie requires a prebaked crust.

2. Blend dry ingredients; with pastry blender or 2 table knives cut in butter until crumbly the size of large peas:
   1¾ cups whole wheat bread flour or pastry flour (p. 19)
      or replace ¼ cup flour with ½ cup toasted wheat germ (p. 15)
   ½ teaspoon salt
   ½ cup cold butter, cut up in pieces, or canola oil (p. 13)

3. Make a well in center, add water, and stir in with a fork just until evenly mixed in (will still be crumbly):
   3 - 4 tablespoons ice water (use 4 Tbsps. with wheat germ)

4. Gather dough together with hands, shaping into a ball in palms of hands, but handling as little as possible.

5. Pat out slightly on wax paper, place another piece wax paper over top and roll out; place in pie pan; trim and flute edges (p. 115).

6. If crust is to be baked before adding filling, prick bottom and sides of crust with fork in several places. Bake in preheated oven at 425° for 8-12 minutes.

<u>Per Recipe</u> *with whole wheat bread flour*
   (does not account for any leftover dough)
   Exchanges: 9.5 Bread, 18 Fat; 1,500 Calories, 26 g protein (7%),
96 g fat (57%; 0 g sugars), 138 g carbohydrate (36%), 26 g dietary fiber,
248 mg cholesterol, 1998 mg sodium, $.85

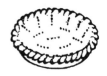

<u>Per serving (wedge) of 8</u> *with whole wheat bread flour* *(does not account for any leftover dough)*
   Exchanges: 1.25 Bread, 2.25 Fat; 188 Calories, 3.5 g protein (7%), 12 g fat (57%),
17 g carbohydrate (36%; 0 g sugars), 1.5 g dietary fiber, 31 mg cholesterol, 250 mg sodium, $.10

For 9" Pie Crust Use recipe above, rolling it out to same thickness as for a 9½" crust. Otherwise it will be too thick. Use the leftover crust for Cinnamon Treat, p. 117.

Whole Wheat Double Pie Crust

A top whole wheat crust is more difficult to handle than a white flour crust and makes the pie quite heavy. I don't make one very often, preferring to top pies with something lighter. See comments on butter and oil under Whole Wheat Single Pie Crust, p. 116, and tips for crusts, p. 115.

AMOUNT: 9½" Pie (For 9" Pie see tip, p. 116)

1. Follow steps #2-4 for single crust, p. 116, using:
   2¼ cups whole wheat bread flour or pastry flour *(p. 19)*
   scant ¾ teaspoon salt
   2/3 cup cold butter, cut up in pieces or canola oil *(p. 13)*
   4-5 tablespoons ice water (add an ice cube for quick cooling)

2. Divide ball of dough, making one piece slightly smaller than the other for the top crust.

3. Roll out bottom crust and fit into pan; add filling. Roll out top crust, lay over filling. Trim edges of crust, pinch together and flute (p. 115).

4. Cut slits or design in top crust to let steam escape. If desired, top leftover dough with cinnamon-sugar and bake for a treat (below).

5. Bake according to chosen pie recipe.

Per Recipe with whole wheat bread flour *(does not account for any leftover dough)*
   Exchanges: 12 Bread, 24 Fat; 1,972 Calories, 34 g protein (7%), 128 g fat (58%),
178 g carbohydrate (36%; 0 g sugars), 34 g dietary fiber, 332 mg cholesterol,
2,676 mg sodium, $1.40

Per serving (wedge) of 8 with whole wheat bread flour *(does not account for any leftover dough)*
   Exchanges: 1.5 Bread, 3 Fat; 247 Calories, 4 g protein (7%), 16 g fat (58%),
22 g carbohydrate (36%; 0 g sugars), 4 g dietary fiber, 42 mg cholesterol, 335 mg sodium, $.20

TOP CRUST VARIATION

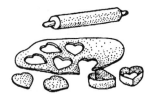

Make small cookie cutter shapes from rolled out top crust; arrange on top of pie filling.

Cinnamon-Sugar Treat   Sprinkle leftover pieces of dough with Cinnamon-Sugar; bake on cookie sheet along with crust or pie for about 10 minutes. For Cinnamon Sugar: blend 5 Tbsps. Sucanat or crystalline fructose with 2 tsps. cinnamon; store in an empty cinnamon jar. Use generously on leftover pie crust dough.

Barley Oat Single Pie Crust

A no wheat pie crust!

AMOUNT: 9" or 9½" Pie

Follow instructions for *Whole Wheat Single Pie Crust*, p. 116, using:
- **1 1/3 cups barley flour** *(from whole grain hulled barley preferred, p. 13)*
- **2/3 cup oat flour** (grind approximately 1 cup rolled oats in blender or ½ cup whole oat groats in flour mill)
- **½ teaspoon salt**
- **1 stick (½ cup) cold butter, cut up in pieces** *(unsalted, p. 32)*
- **3 tablespoons cold water**

Per serving (wedge) of 8
Exchanges: 2 Bread, 2.25 Fat; 228 Calories, 5 g protein (8%), 12.5 g fat (50%), 23 g carbohydrate (41%; 0 g sugars), 3 g dietary fiber, 31 mg cholesterol, 139 mg sodium, $.15

Sue's Special Rice Pie Crust

No wheat! Delicately crisp, this crust is especially good with Lemon Tofu Cheese Pie, p. 124, or Pumpkin Pie, p. 127.

AMOUNT: 9½" Pie
Bake 350° for About 20 minutes

1. Preheat oven to 350° if pie requires prebaked crust.

2. Blend flour and salt; with pastry blender or 2 table knives cut in butter until crumbly the size of large peas:
   - **1½ cups brown rice flour** *(p. 14)*
   - **½ teaspoon salt**
   - **½ stick (¼ cup) cold butter, cut up in pieces** *(unsalted, p. 32)*

3. Make a well in center, add juice, and stir in with a fork just until evenly mixed in:
   - **½ cup cold pineapple or orange juice**

4. Place dough in pie pan; let rest 10 minutes.

5. With flour on fingers, shape dough into pie pan pressing into sides of pan first; flute edges (p. 115).

6. For prebaked crust, prick bottom and sides with fork in several places.

7. Bake in preheated oven at 350° about 20 minutes or until golden, or leave unbaked if called for in pie recipe.

Per serving (wedge) of 8
Exchanges: 1.25 Bread, 1 Fat, 0.25 Fruit; 141 Calories, 2 g protein (5%), 6 g fat (39%), 20 g carbohydrate (56%; 2 g sugars), 1.5 g dietary fiber, 16 mg cholesterol, 136 mg sodium, $.10

Graham Cracker Crust

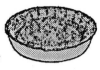

My choice of whole grain graham crackers for good taste are Mi-Del or New Morning brand (p. 13). See tip for making cracker crumbs below.

AMOUNT: 9" or 9½" Pie
Bake 350° for 10 minutes

1. Preheat oven to 350°.

2. Blend together:
   1½ cups whole wheat graham cracker crumbs *(p. 13; see below)*
   (1 packet of 7 double crackers)
   2 tablespoons crystalline fructose *(p. 13)* **or Sucanat** *(p. 14)*
   1/3 cup melted butter *(unsalted preferred, p. 32)*

3. Press firmly and evenly into sides and bottom of pie pan.

4. Bake in preheated oven at 350° for 10 minutes or follow variation below.

5. Cool before adding filling.

<u>Per Recipe</u>
Exchanges: 9 Bread, 12 Fat; 1,262 Calories, 9.5 g protein (3%), 70 g fat (54%), 124 g carbohydrate (43%; 46 g sugars), 9 g dietary fiber, 166 mg cholesterol, 1,178 mg sodium, $1.25

<u>Per serving (wedge) of 8</u>
Exchanges: 1.25 Bread, 1.5 Fat; 158 Calories, 1 g. protein (3%), 9 g. fat (54%), 15.5 g carbohydrate (43%; 6 g sugars), 1 g dietary fiber, 21 mg cholesterol, 147 mg sodium, $.15

<u>Per serving (square) of 9</u> *from an 8" or 9" square pan*
Exchanges: 1 Bread, 1.25 Fat, 140 Calories, 1 g protein (3%), 8 g fat (54%), 14 g carbohydrate (43%; 5 g sugars), 1 g dietary fiber, 18 mg cholesterol, 131 mg sodium, $.15

VARIATION

Do not bake crust. Place in freezer for 10 minutes or longer. Crust will not hold together quite as well. I use this method for an 8" or 9" square pan, as for *Yogurt Pie*, p. 128 (yogurt filling helps hold the crust together).

Graham Cracker Crumbs: To make cracker crumbs, break them up with your hands as you place them inside a plastic bag, away from the open end. Lay bag flat on counter without closing it at the top (If closed, air gets trapped inside and the bag may pop a hole as crackers are being crushed). With rolling pin crush the broken crackers, redistributing as necessary to crush evenly. One packet of double crackers makes about 1½ cups crumbs crushed in this way. Crackers may also be crushed in blender, but are harder to crush evenly without crushing them too finely, and it's messier.

Fresh Apple Pie

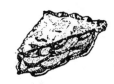

See tip for selecting baking apples, p. 131.

AMOUNT: 9" or 9½ Pie
Bake 425° for About 50 minutes

1. Prepare choice of **single or double pie crust, unbaked** (pp. 116-18). Preheat oven to 425°.

2. Blend first 4 ingredients; drizzle 1/3 over bottom of pie crust; add apples and top with remaining sugar-flour mixture:
   ½ - ¾ cup honey or crystalline fructose *(p. 13)*
   2 tablespoons whole wheat or whole wheat pastry flour *(p. 14)*
   1 teaspoon cinnmon
   1 teaspoon lemon or orange peel *(see tip, p. 106)*
   8 cups peeled apple slices (8-10 medium apples)

3. Add top crust, if desired (steps #3, 4, p. 117); bake in preheated oven at 425° for about 50 minutes until crust is golden and apples tender.

Per serving of 8, filling only (see Fat % Chart, pp. 35-38 for fat % with choice of crust)
   Exchanges: 1 Fruit; 137 Calories, 35 g carbohydrate (98%; 33 g sugars),
2.5 g dietary fiber, 1 mg sodium, $.25

Fresh Berry or Cherry Pie

AMOUNT: 9½" Pie
Bake 450° for 10 minutes; 350° for 20-30 minutes

1. Prepare choice of **single or double pie crust, unbaked** (pp. 116-18). Preheat oven to 450°.

2. Mix ingredients together except butter; pour into unbaked pie crust and dot with butter:
   4 cups fresh berries or pitted pie cherries
   3 tablespoons quick-cooking tapioca *(p 15)*
      or 1/3 cup whole wheat flour or pastry flour *(p 14)*
   ½ - ¾ cup honey or crystalline fructose *(p. 13)*
   ½ teaspoon cinnamon
   1½ tablespoons soft butter *(unsalted preferred, p. 32)*

3. Add top crust, if desired (steps #3, 4, p. 117); bake in preheated oven at 450° for 10 minutes; reduce heat to 350° and bake 20-30 minutes longer.

Per serving of 8, filling only with fresh blueberries and tapioca
   (see Fat % Chart, pp. 35-38 for fat % with choice of crust)
   Exchanges: 0.25 Bread, 0.5 Fat, 0.75 Fruit; 138 Calories, 0.5 g protein (2%), 2.5 g. fat (16%),
31 g carbohydrate (84%; 25 g sugars), 2 g dietary fiber, 6 mg cholesterol, 6 mg sodium, $.35

Heavenly Pecan Chip Pie

Another gourmet dessert from Judy Phillips (p. 72). Serve slightly warm or at room temperature, with Whipped Cream (p. 155) or Whipped Topping (p. 159), if desired. It's great cold, too! Carob Chips are especially tasty in this recipe.

AMOUNT: 9" or 9½" Pie
Bake 325° for 50-60 minutes

1. Prepare choice of **single pie crust, unbaked** (pp. 116-18).

2. Preheat oven to 325°.

	9" Pie	**9½" Pie**
3. Melt over very low heat; set aside to cool until ready to use: **butter** *(unsalted preferred, p. 32)*	¼ cup	1/3 cup
4. Sprinkle over bottom of crust: **chopped pecans**	1¼ cups	1½ cups
carob chips *(p. 13)*	1 cup	1¼ cups
5. Whisk together eggs, honey, and vanilla; blend in butter: **large eggs**	3	4
honey	1 cup	1¼ cups
vanilla	½ teaspoon	¾ teaspoon
butter, melted, slightly cooled		

6. Pour egg mixture into pie shell. This will not seem full enough, but it will rise up during baking.

7. Bake in preheated oven at 325° for 50-60 minutes or until firm.

8. Store leftover pie in refrigerator (p. 58).

Per serving of 8 - 9" pie, filling only (see Fat % Chart, pp. 35-38 for fat % with choice of crust)
   Exchanges: 0.5 Meat, 1 Bread, 4.75 Fat; 443 Calories, 6.5 g protein (6%), 28 g fat (52%), 50 g carbohydrate (43%; 45 g sugars), 1.5 g dietary fiber, 95 mg cholesterol, 29 mg sodium, $.90

Per serving of 8 - 9½" pie, filling only
   Exchanges: 0.75 Meat, 1.25 Bread, 6 Fat; 554 Calories, 8 g protein (6%), 33.5 g fat (52%), 62.5 g carbohydrate (43%; 56 g sugars), 1.5 g dietary fiber, 127 mg cholesterol, 38 mg sodium, $1.10

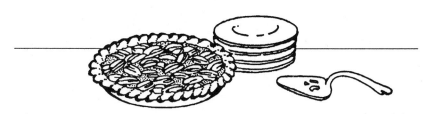

Banana Cream Pie

Churn up your digestive system and emotions by reviewing a few frozen pie ingredients labels in the supermarket. Then come home and make one of your own with real wholesome food ingredients!

AMOUNT: 9½" Pie*

1. Prepare choice of **single pie crust, baked** (pp. 116-119).

2. Prepare hot *Vanilla Pudding,* p. 137, increasing the ingredient amounts to the following:
   - **3 cups cold nonfat milk** *(or alternative, p. 39)*
   - **4½ tablespoons cornstarch or arrowroot powder** *(p. 13)*
   - **½ cup crystalline fructose** *(p. 13)* **or 3/8 cup honey**
   - **3/8 teaspoon salt**
   - **3 slightly beaten egg yolks** (reserve whites for meringue)
   - **3 tablespoons butter** *(unsalted preferred, p. 32)*
   - **1½ teaspoons vanilla**

3. Fold bananas into pudding and pour into crust: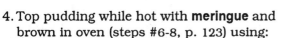
   - **2 sliced bananas, peeled**

4. Top pudding while hot with **meringue** and brown in oven (steps #6-8, p. 123) using:
   - **3 egg whites** (leftover from pudding recipe)
   - **1 teaspoon lemon juice**
   - **3 tablespoons crystalline fructose** *(p. 13)*

5. Chill thoroughly. Store leftover pie in refrigerator (p. 58).

*Note For a 9" pie, in step #2 do not increase *Vanilla Pudding* recipe on p. 137, except cornstarch. Increase cornstarch from 2 Tbsps. to 3 Tbsps.

Per serving of 8, filling only with meringue (see Fat % Chart, pp. 35-38 for fat % with choice of crust)
  Exchanges: 0.5 Meat, 0.5 Milk, 0.25 Bread, 1 Fat, 0.5 Fruit; 213 Calories, 6 g protein (11%), 7 g fat (28%), 33.5 g carbohydrate (61%; 30 g sugars), 1 g dietary fiber, 93 mg. cholesterol, 27 mg sodium, $.35

VARIATIONS

In place of meringue, top pie with:
   - **½ cup toasted medium shred coconut, unsweetened** *(p. 13)*
     or ½ cup toasted finely chopped almonds or sliced almonds
     (toast coconut at 350° for 5-8 minutes just until lightly browned; to toast almonds, see p. 73)

Per serving of 8, with filling only, with coconut
  Exchanges: 0.5 Meat, 0.5 Milk, 0.25 Bread, 1.5 Fat, 0.5 Fruit; 221 Calories, 6 g protein (11%), 9 g fat (37%), 30 g carbohydrate (52%; 30 g sugars), 2 g dietary fiber, 93 mg cholesterol, 29 mg sodium, $.35

Lemon Meringue Pie

Lemon Meringue Pie has always been my favorite.

AMOUNT: 9" or 9½" Pie

	9" Pie	9½" Pie
1. Prepare choice of **single pie crust, baked** (pp. 116-119).		
2. Separate **large eggs** (p. 53).	**3**	**4**

3. In saucepan mix dry ingredients; gradually whisk in water, bring to boil; whisk constantly until thickened and clear, about 1 minute:

	9" Pie	9½" Pie
cornstarch *(p.13)*	**1/3 cup**	**½ cup**
crystalline fructose *(p. 13)*	**¾ cup**	**1 1/8 cups**
cold water (room temperature)	**1½ cups**	**2¼ cups**

4. Whisk part of the thickened mixture into **beaten egg yolks.** Blend mixture with egg back into remaining mixture in saucepan. Return to boil 1 minute, whisking constantly.

5. Remove from heat; stir in and pour into crust:

	9" Pie	9½" Pie
butter *(unsalted preferred, p. 32)*	**3 Tbsps.**	**¼ cup**
lemon juice (fresh preferred)	**¼ cup**	**6 Tbsps.**
grated lemon peel *(see tip, p. 106)*	**1 Tbsp.**	**4 tsps.**

6. **Meringue**--Beat egg whites with lemon juice on high speed in mixer until frothy; gradually add fructose until stiff peaks form, but not dry (p. 53):

	9" Pie	9½" Pie
egg whites	**3**	**4**
lemon juice	**1 tsp.**	**1½ tsps.**
crystalline fructose	**3 Tbsps.**	**¼ cup**

7. Pile meringue on top of hot lemon filling, sealing it to the edge of the pie crust. Swirl meringue to make peaks.

8. Bake in preheated oven at 400° for about 5 minutes until meringue is lightly browned (browns quickly). Cool and chill. Store leftover pie in refrigerator (p. 58).

Per serving of 8 - 9" pie filling only with meringue
(see Fat % Chart, pp. 35-38 for fat % with choice of crust)
Exchanges:0.5 Meat, 0.25 Bread, 1 Fat; 179 Calories, 2.5 g protein (5%),
6.5 g fat (32%), 29 g carbohydrate (63%; 24 g sugars), 92 mg cholesterol, 26 mg sodium, $.25

Per serving of 8 - 9½" pie, filling only with meringue
(see Fat % Chart, pp. 35-38 for fat % with choice of crust)
Exchanges: 0.5 Meat, 0.5 Bread, 1.5 Fat; 254 Calories, 3 g protein (5%),
8.5 g fat (30%), 42.5 g carbohydrate (65%; 35 g sugars), 122 mg cholesterol, 35 mg sodium, $.35

Lemon Tofu Cheese Pie

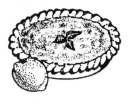

Creamy and delicate in flavor, this pie is lower in fat and calories and higher in protein than the traditional cheese cake. Dress it up with fruit topping or serve it plain.

AMOUNT: 9½" Pie

1. Prepare choice of **single pie crust, baked** (pp. 116-119).

2. Drain tofu on plate between double thickness of paper towels at least 30 minutes:
   16 oz. block tofu, soft or regular *(p. 15)*

3. In small saucepan whisk gelatine into milk and let stand 5 minutes to soften; bring just barely to a boil over moderately low heat, whisking constantly, to dissolve gelatine:
   1/3 cup cold lowfat milk *(or alternative, p. 39)*
   2 envelopes (4 teaspoons) unflavored gelatine *(p. 15)*

4. With electric mixer blend in each ingredient in order given (mixture will not be completely smooth):
   8 oz. light cream cheese or cream cheese, softened
   crumbled tofu, well drained
   ½ cup honey
   2 tablespoons lemon peel *(see tip, p. 106)*
   2 tablespoons lemon juice (fresh preferred)
   1 teaspoon vanilla
   ¼ teaspoon salt
   dissolved gelatine-milk mixture

5 Puree mixture in blender, 2 cups at a time, until completely smooth.

6. Pour mixture into pie crust; chill until set.

7. Optional--Spread evenly over top of pie:
   20 oz. can crushed pineapple, unsweetened, drained
   mint leaves (for garnish, if available)

8. Store leftover pie in refrigerator (p. 58).

Per serving of 8, filling only, with crushed pineapple topping
   (see Fat % Chart, pp. 35-38 for fat % with choice of crust)
   Exchanges: 0.5 Meat, 1.75 Fat, 0.75 Fruit; 210 Calories, 8.5 g protein (16%), 8.5 g fat (35%), 27.5 g carbohydrate (50%; 27 g sugars), 0.5 g dietary fiber, 23 mg cholesterol, 192 mg sodium, $.75

Carob Tofu Pie

A tasty variation of Lemon Tofu Cheese Pie.

AMOUNT: 9½" Pie

1. Prepare **Coconut Almond Pie Crust** (below).
2. Use recipe for **Lemon Tofu Cheese Pie**, p. 124, with following changes in step #4:
   omit lemon juice and lemon peel
   increase to 1½ teaspoons vanilla
   blend in **6 tablespoons carob powder** *(p. 13)*
      (stir through strainer to remove lumps)
3. Optional--Before chilling pie top with:
   ½ cup toasted medium shred coconut, unsweetened *(p. 13)*
      (Toast coconut at 350° on a cookie sheet for 5-8 minutes
      to brown lightly)
4. Store leftover pie in refrigerator (p. 58).

Per serving of 8, filling only, coconut topping not included (for fat % with crust see p. 38)
Exchanges:0.5 Meat, 0.5 Bread, 1.75 Fat; 204 Calories, 9 g protein (17%), 8.5 g fat (35%),
25.5 g carbohydrate (48%; 19 g sugars), 0.5 g dietary fiber, 23 mg cholesterol, 257 mg sodium, $.55

Coconut Almond Single Pie Crust

Rich and yummy! Yes, I know--it's high fat, too!

AMOUNT: 9" or 9½" Pie
Bake at 300° for 20 minutes, or Chill

1. To bake (see step #5), preheat oven to 300°.
2. Finely grind almonds in blender; mix with coconut in mixing bowl:
   ½ cup almonds, unsalted, unroasted *(p. 43)*
   1½ cups macaroon shred coconut, unsweetened *(p. 13)*
      (sliced coconut can be blended in blender for this if
      macaroon shred is not on hand)
3. Blend in thoroughly:
   5 tablespoons (½ stick + 1 Tbsp.) melted unsalted butter
4. Pour mixture into pie pan; press into sides of pan first with
   fingers. With fork lightly spread and press mixture evenly
   into bottom of pan (fingers don't work very well for this).
5. Bake in preheated oven at 300° for 20 minutes or chill in
   freezer until firm.

Per serving (1 wedge) of 8
Exchanges: 0.25 Meat, 0.25 Bread, 3.5 Fat; 193 Calories, 2.5 g protein (5%), 19 g fat (86%),
5 g carbohydrate (9%; 0 g sugars), 4.5 g dietary fiber, 19 mg cholesterol, 5 mg sodium, $.20

Quick Coconut Blender Pie

You won't believe this tasty and intriguing pie. Made in less than 5 minutes, it forms its own "crust", top and bottom, during baking! Don't shun coconut because of its fat content. It is a good food (1 Timothy 4:4-5), important in the tropics for thousands of years (see p. 94).

AMOUNT: 9½" Pie   **Bake at 350° for 60 minutes**

> **Note:** In this recipe you can use either unmilled grain or flour (see tip below). Follow step #1 carefully to use the right blending procedure for the one or the other.

1. To use unmilled grain, place it in blender with milk; blend on high speed for 3-4 minutes; briefly blend in remaining ingredients. To use flour, put everything together in blender and blend briefly:

   2 cups lowfat milk or *Better Than Milk Tofu Beverage* (p. 39)
   1/3 cup your choice of whole grain, uncooked (see Tip below)
      or ½ cup whole grain flour (see Tip below; pp. 13-14)
   3 eggs
   ¼ cup butter (room temperature) **or canola oil** (p. 13)
   ½ cup mild-flavored honey (p. 25) **or crystalline fructose** (p. 13)
   ¼ teaspoon salt
   1 teaspoon vanilla
   1 cup macaroon coconut, unsweetened (p. 42)
   1 oz. bottle (scant 3 Tbsps.) coconut extract
   1 teaspoon grated lemon, lime, or orange peel, optional
   ½ teaspoon baking powder (low sodium or Rumford preferred, p. 13)

2. Pour into greased pie pan and bake at 350° for 60 minutes or until knife comes clean out of center. Pie will be puffed up, but will settle down. Serve slightly warm or chilled. Refrigerate leftover pie.

Per serving of 8 with lowfat milk, brown rice flour, butter, honey
   Exchanges: 0.5 Meat, 0.25 Milk, 0.5 Bread, 2.25 Fat; 254 Calories, 5.5 g protein (8%), 14 g fat (48%), 28.5 g carbohydrate (43%; 20 g sugars), 3 g dietary fiber, 100 mg cholesterol, 185 mg sodium, $.60

Per serving of 8 with Better Than Milk Tofu Beverage, pastry wheat flour, canola oil, fructose
   Exchanges: 0.5 Meat, 0.75 Bread, 2.5 Fat; 244 Calories, 4 g protein (7%), 15.5 g fat (55%), 24.5 g carbohydrate (38%; 13 g sugars), 3.5 g dietary fiber, 80 mg cholesterol, 126 mg sodium, $.60

> **About Grains:** I have made this blender pie successfully with 4 grains: brown rice, millet, Kamut, and whole wheat pastry grain. My favorite is with millet, but we like them all. With whole wheat pastry flour, the top crust is a little thicker and darker than the others. When grain is milled into flour, 1/3 cup grain makes about ½ cup flour. I prefer using the grain over flour for maximum nutritional value and flavor.

Pumpkin Pie

Whenever I make the filling for this pie, I use the entire can of 2 cups pumpkin. This makes more filling than will fit in some pie pans. Put extra filling in a baking dish and bake it along with the pie for a very tasty Pumpkin Pudding. Our daughter Sharon actually prefers the filling as a pudding without the crust! Scant means a little less than the full amount.

AMOUNT: 9" or 9½" Pie
Bake 375° about 45 minutes

1. Prepare choice of **single pie crust, unbaked** (pp. 116-118).

2. Preheat oven to 375°.

3. Blend thoroughly in blender:

    1 lb. can (2 cups) pumpkin or fresh pumpkin *(see cooking tip below)*
    1 1/3 cups lowfat milk *(or alternative, p. 39)*
    4 eggs
    scant ½ cup honey
    scant 1½ teaspoons cinnamon
    scant ¾ teaspoon ground ginger
    scant ¾ teaspoon nutmeg
    ½ teaspoon salt
    scant 1½ teaspoons vanilla

4. Pour filling into unbaked pie crust until reasonably full. Pour extra filling into a greased oven-proof bowl.

5. Bake in preheated oven at 375° for about 45 minutes until set. Do not expect it to be totally firm in center. It will set more as it cools.

6. Serve with whipped cream, if desired. Keep refrigerated (p. 58).

Per serving of 8, filling only (see Fat % Chart, pp. 35-38 for fat % with choice of crust)
 Exchanges: 0.5 Meat, 0.25 Milk, 0.25 Bread, 0.25 Fat; 147 Calories, 5 g protein (13%), 4 g fat (22%), 25 g carbohydrate (65%; 19 g sugars), 1 g dietary fiber, 110 mg cholesterol, 195 mg sodium, $.40

REDUCED FAT VARIATION

Use **nonfat milk** and **8 unbeaten egg whites** in place of eggs. Add **¼ cup nonfat non-instant dry milk powder** (p. 14).

Per serving of 8, filling only (see Fat % Chart, pp. 35-38 for fat % with choice of crust)
 Exchanges: 0.25 Meat, 0.25 Milk, 0.25 Bread; 131 Calories, 6.5 g protein (19%), 0.5 g fat (2%), 27 g carbohydrate (79%; 23 g sugars), 1 g dietary fiber, 2 mg cholesterol, 210 mg sodium, $.50

Cooking Fresh Pumpkin: Cut unpeeled pumpkin in large chunks; place upside down over boiling water in steamer basket or on rack in a wok. Steam until tender, about 30 minutes. Cool; scrape pulp out of skin. Freeze in desired portions.

Yogurt Pie

One of our daughter Sharon's favorite desserts, this light, easy-to-make pie, is served at our Taste 'n Tell Workshop luncheon. The coconut variation is delicious. I prefer to make it in a square pan, but it can be made just as well in a 9" pie pan. For a 9½" pie, use Graham Cracker Crust recipe, p.119.

AMOUNT: 8"-9" Pan or 9" Pie (8-9 Servings)

1. For graham cracker crust blend together;
   1 cup graham cracker crumbs *(p. 13, see tip, p. 119)*
   (about 5 crackers)
   1 tablespoon crystalline fructose *(preferred, p. 13)*
   or 2 tablespoons *Sucanat* **or date sugar**
   ¼ cup (½ stick) melted butter *(unsalted preferred, p. 32)*

2. Pat crumbs in bottom of 8" or 9" square pan; chill in freezer at least 10-12 minutes.

3. In small saucepan whisk gelatine into juice; let stand 5 minutes to soften; heat to boiling while stirring with whisk until gelatin is dissolved; stir in honey:
   juice drained from 8 oz. can crushed pineapple, unsweetened
   (set the drained pineapple aside)
   2 envelopes (4 teaspoons) unflavored gelatine *(p. 15)*
   ¼ cup honey

4. Whisk together thoroughly in mixing bowl; pour into graham cracker crust; chill until set:
   3 cups nonfat or lowfat plain yogurt *(or pasteurized alternative, p. 39)*
   1½ teaspoons vanilla
   reserved crushed pineapple
   dissolved gelatine-honey mixture
   ½ cup medium shred coconut, unsweetened, optional *(p. 13)*
   ½ teaspoon coconut extract, optional (add with coconut)

5. Optional--Score into servings; garnish each, as desired, with:
   ½ fresh strawberry
   2 half-slices kiwi fruit

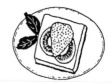

6. Store leftover pie in refrigerator (p. 58).

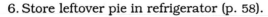

Per serving of 9 from 8" or 9" square pan, with nonfat yogurt; coconut, garnish not included
    Exchanges: 0.25 Milk, 0.75 Bread, 1 Fat, 0.25 Fruit; 179 Calories, 6.5 g protein (15%), 9 g fat (30%), 25 g carbohydrate (56%; 20 g sugars), 1 g dietary fiber, 15 mg cholesterol, 133 mg sodium, $.45

Per serving of 8 from 9" pie pan, with nonfat yogurt; coconut, garnish not included
    Exchanges: 0.5 Milk, 0.75 Bread, 1.25 Fat, 0.25 Fruit; 201 Calories, 7.5 g protein (15%), 6.5 g fat (30%), 28 g carbohydrate (56%; 22 g sugars), 1 g dietary fiber, 28 mg cholesterol, 152 mg sodium, $.50

Puddings
& Desserts

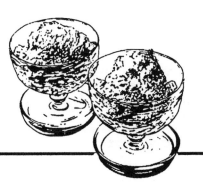

She speaks with wisdom, and faithful instruction is on her tongue.
She watches over the affairs of her household and does not eat the
bread of idleness.
Proverbs 31:27

Puddings & Desserts

Apple or Peach Crisp

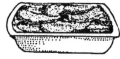

This is a revised Betty Crocker recipe. Delicious served with milk, yogurt, or whipped cream. For extra fiber and nutrients leave apples unpeeled, or use a good cleaner on waxed apples (see tip below). An unpeeled apple has more than twice the fiber of a peeled apple.

AMOUNT: 6 Servings
Bake 375° for 30-35 minutes, uncovered

1. Preheat oven to 375°. Grease or spray an 8"-10" baking pan or 1½ qt. casserole dish generously with non-stick spray (p. 54).

2. Place in pan or casserole dish:
   4 cups sliced baking apples (about 6 medium),
   peeled, cored *(see Apple Selections for Baking below)*
   or peeled sliced fresh peaches

3. Blend until crumbly; spread evenly over fruit slices:
   ½ cup whole wheat pastry flour *(p. 14; or alternative, pp. 20-22)*
   ½ cup Quick or Old Fashioned Quaker Oats, uncooked
   ¼ cup crystalline fructose *(p. 13)* **or ½ cup Sucanat** *(p. 14)*
   ¾ teaspoon cinnamon
   ¾ teaspoon nutmeg
   1/3 cup soft butter *(unsalted preferred, p. 32)*

4. Bake uncovered in preheated oven at 375° for 30-45 minutes or until apples are tender.

Per serving of 6 - Apple Crisp
 Exchanges: 1 Bread, 2 Fat, 0.75 Fruit; 235 Calories, 2.5 g protein (5%), 11 g fat (41%), 34 g carbohydrate (55%; 19 g sugars), 3.5 g dietary fiber, 28 mg cholesterol, 2 mg sodium, $.25

Per serving of 6 - Peach Crisp
 Exchanges: 1 Bread, 2 Fat, 0.75 Fruit; 230 Calories, 3 g protein (5%), 11.5 g fat (42%), 33 g carbohydrate (53%; 16 g sugars), 3 g dietary fiber, 28 mg cholesterol, 3 mg sodium, $.40

Apple Selections for Baking: Apples vary in tartness and juiciness. Varieties that are more suitable for baking are Roman Beauty, Rhode Island Greening, Northern Spy, York Imperial, Winesap, Cortland, Granny Smith, Gravenstein, and Pippin. Better eaten raw are Jonathan, Macintosh, and Red Delicious.

Wax Removal: Completely removing wax from apples is difficult. *Dr. Donsbach's Superoxy Food Wash* (containing water, hydrogen peroxide, and a special grapefruit seed extract) available at health food stores, is advertized to help remove waxes, and reduce pesticide, herbicide, and fungicide residues on most fruits and vegetables.

Baked Apples

Try these for a special breakfast treat, as well as for dessert. See tips for apple selection and wax removal, p. 131. Prepare for baking in advance or the evening before, covering prepared apples with plastic wrap; refrigerate. Pop in the oven an hour before serving. Delicious with plain yogurt or milk over the top.

AMOUNT: 6 Servings
Bake 375° for about 45 minutes, uncovered

1. Preheat oven to 375°.

2. **Make Syrup** In a small saucepan whisk together all but lemon juice, bring just to a boil, lower heat and simmer 5 minutes; remove from heat and stir in the lemon juice:
   1½ cups water
   ¼ cup honey or crystalline fructose *(p. 13)*
   2 tablespoons butter *(unsalted preferred, p. 32)*
   ¼ teaspoon cinnamon
   1 tablespoon lemon juice

3. Chop nuts and raisins together until fairly fine with a chef's knife (p. 49); blend with fructose and cinnamon:
   3 tablespoons walnuts
   3 tablespoons raisins
   2 tablespoons crystalline fructose
   1½ teaspoons cinnamon

4. Wash and core apples; with a small sharp paring knife make small shallow cuts around cored edges of apples at the top:
   6 baking apples *(see tips for selection and wax removal, p. 131)*

5. Set apples in an 8" or 9" baking dish. Fill apple cavities with the **nut-raisin mixture**. Dot each apple with:
   about ¼ teaspoon butter

6. Pour **hot syrup** (step #2) in bottom of baking dish.

7. Bake uncovered in preheated oven at 375° for about 45 minutes or until apples are tender; baste a couple of times with the hot syrup during baking.

8. Serve in cereal bowl with syrup.

Per serving of 6, with syrup evenly divided, large (7½ oz.) apples
Exchanges: 1.25 Fat, 1.5 Fruit; 216 Calories, 1.5 g protein (3%), 7 g fat (27%),
41.5 g carbohydrate (71%; 43 g sugars), 4 g dietary fiber, 12 mg cholesterol, 8 mg sodium, $.30

Judy's Apple Crisp

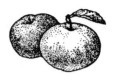

Rich! Serve for a delicious company dessert with cheddar cheese slices and herb tea.

AMOUNT: 9" - 10" Pie Pan
Bake Crust only: 350° for 10 minutes

1. Preheat oven to 350°.

2. Mix together:
   2 cups favorite granola or *Simple Granola* (*Breakfasts, p. 116*)
   1/3 cup melted butter (*unsalted preferred, p. 32*)

3. Reserve **¼ cup granola mixture** for topping. Press remaining mixture into bottom of pie pan; bake at 350° for 10 minutes; cool.

4. In blender blend until smooth; pour into cooled crust:
   8 oz. light cream cheese, *Neufchatel,* or cream cheese
   1 cup nonfat yogurt (*p. 39*)

5. Core and thinly slice apples; cook in a very small amount of water until just tender:
   4-5 baking apples, unpeeled
   (*see tips for Apple Selections and Wax Removal, p. 131*)

6. Remove apples from heat, drain; mix in:
   ¼ cup honey
   ½ teaspoon cinnamon
   dash ground cloves

7. Spread apples over cheese-yogurt filling; top with:
   reserved granola mixture.

8. Chill 3 hours.

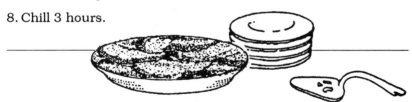

Per serving of 8, with light cream cheese, 5 medium apples, Simple Granola
   Exchanges: 0.25 Milk, 1.25 Bread, 3.75 Fat, 0.75 Fruit; 364 Calories, 8.5 g protein (9%), 19 g fat (46%), 43 g carbohydrate (45%; 28 g sugars), 4 g dietary fiber, 43 mg cholesterol, 133 mg. sodium, $.55

Per serving of 8, with cream cheese, 5 medium apples, Simple Granola
   Exchanges: 0.25 Milk, 1.25 Bread, 4.5 Fat, 1.25 Fruit; 416 Calories, 8 g protein (7%), 23 g fat (47%), 50 g carbohydrate (46%; 28 g sugars), 4.5 g dietary fiber, 52 mg cholesterol, 104 mg.sodium,$.50

Fruit Cobbler

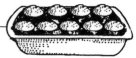

A tasty quick way to use an abundance of fresh fruit in season. Serve warm with milk or whipped cream.

AMOUNT: 8 Servings
Bake 400° for 25-30 minutes, uncovered

1. Preheat oven to 400°.

2. In saucepan blend dry ingredients and gradually whisk in water or fruit juice; bring to boil, stirring constantly with whisk until clear and thickened:
   1/3 cup honey or crystalline fructose *(p. 13)*
   1 tablespoon cornstarch or arrowroot powder *(p. 13)*
   1 cup water
   (with canned fruit use the drained juice + water as needed)

3. Remove from heat; in 1½ qt. casserole dish fold into:
   3 cups sliced fresh fruit *(see tips, p. 131)*
      or 2½ cups canned fruit *(packed in its own juice, p. 39)*
   (peaches, apricots, apples, berries, pitted pie cherries)

4. Dot with **1 tablespoon butter** and sprinkle with **cinnamon.**

5. In a separate bowl blend together:
   1 cup whole wheat pastry flour *(p. 14; or alternative, pp. 20-22)*
   2 teaspoons crystalline fructose
   1½ teaspoons baking powder *(low sodium or Rumford preferred, p. 13)*
   ½ teaspoon salt

6. With a pastry blender (p. 49), or 2 table knives cut butter into flour mixture to make crumbly meal the size of small peas; stir into the milk just until mixed (do not overmix):
   3 tablespoons soft butter *(unsalted preferred, p. 32)*
   ½ cup nonfat milk *(or alternative, p. 39)*

7. Drop dough by spoonfuls over hot fruit.

8. Bake uncovered in preheated oven at 400° for 25-30 minutes or until fruit is tender.

Per serving of 8 <u>with fresh peaches</u>
Exchanges: 1 Bread, 1.25 Fat, 0.25 Fruit; 188 Calories, 2.5 g protein (5%), 6.5 g fat (28%), 34 g carboydrate (66%; 18 g sugars), 2.5 g dietary fiber, 16 mg cholesterol, 136 mg sodium, $.25

Per serving of 8 <u>with fresh apples</u>
Exchanges: 1 Bread, 1.25 Fat, 0.5 Fruit; 193 Calories, 2.5 g protein (5%), 6 g fat (27%), 35 g carbohydrate (68%; 19 g sugars), 2.5 g dietary fiber, 16 mg cholesterol, 136 mg sodium, $.20

Dessert Crepes

Crepes are very thin pancakes that are fun and easy to make with a variety of fillings and toppings. I make crepes in the same pans I reserve for omelets (see **Breakfasts**, p. 145, for purchasing and seasoning an omelet or crepe pan). Use a 6"-8" pan with curved sides. With 2 pans you can turn these out in about 10 minutes. Leftover crepes freeze well; to freeze, wrap snuggly in plastic wrap, then foil.

AMOUNT: 8-9 Crepes in 8" Pan (4 Servings)

1. Place ingredients in blender; if using flour, blend 30 seconds; if using grain, blend 3-5 minutes (see note below):
   - **1 egg or 2 egg whites**
   - **¾ cup nonfat milk** (or alternative, p. 39)
   - **1½ teaspoons oil** (canola oil preferred, p. 13)
   - **3/16 teaspoon salt** (1/8 tsp. + half 1/8 tsp.)
   - **1½ teaspoons honey**
   - **¼ teaspoon cinnamon**
   - **½ cup flour or 1/3 cup whole grain (raw, uncooked)***
     Kamut, whole wheat pastry, spelt, or other grain (p. 13)

2. Add **½ teaspoon olive oil** to moderately hot crepe or omelet pan before baking each 2 crepes, **or spray as needed** with olive oil non-stick spray to prevent sticking.

3. Pour **3 Tbsps. batter** (a ¼ cup measure ¾ full) into hot pan; quickly tilt pan to swirl the batter evenly to edges of the pan.

> **Batter Tip:** The flour in the batter tends to settle to the bottom quickly; briefly reblend it before making each crepe by turning on blender, or pour the batter into a mixing bowl and stir it up each time with a spoon or with the ¼ measure as you are filling it for the next crepe.

4. Cook until browned on edges, about 1-2 minutes; loosen with pancake turner and flip over; cook lightly on reverse side.

5. Stack on plate until ready to fill and fold or roll.

6. Complete crepes with choice of filling and topping, pp. 136-37.

Per crepe of 8 with Kamut flour
   Exchanges: 0.25 Meat, 0.5 bread, 0.5 Fat; 80 Calories, 3 g protein (15%), 4 g fat (43%), 8.5 g carbohydrate (41%; 2 g sugars), 0.5 g dietary fiber, 27 mg cholesterol, 59 mg sodium, $.10

*The idea of putting whole grain, unmilled and uncooked, into the blender with liquid ingredients is such a new concept to most people. They really don't believe I mean what the recipe says. See **Breakfasts**, p. 82, *Whole Grain Blender Magic.*

Apple Walnut Crepes

AMOUNT: 8-9 Crepes (4 Servings--2 Each)

1. Make *Dessert Crepes*, p. 135.

2. In fry pan cook apples in butter over low heat until tender; stir in walnuts and cinnamon sugar:
   2 tablespoons melted butter *(unsalted preferred, p. 32)*
   4 small or 3 medium apples, peeled, thinly sliced *(see tips, p. 131)*
   ½ cup chopped walnuts
   8 teaspoons cinnamon sugar *(see p. 115)*

3. Place 2-3 tablespoons apple filling on one side of crepe; roll up and place seam side down on serving plate.

4. If desired briefly warm rolled crepes in 300°-350° oven, uncovered.

5. To serve, top crepes with:
   leftover apple filling
   whipped cream

Per 1 filled crepe of 8; whipped cream not included
*   Exchanges: 0.25 Meat, 0.5 Bread, 2 Fat, 0.5 Fruit; 186 Calories, 5 g protein (11%), 11.5 g fat (52%), 18 g carbohydrate (37%; 12 g sugars), 1.5 g dietary fiber, 35 mg cholesterol, 60 mg sodium, $.25*

VARIATION
Fill and top crepes with *Dried Apple Topping,* **Breakfasts,** p. 220.

Lemon Fruit Crepes

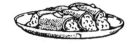

AMOUNT: 8-9 Crepes (4 Servings--2 Each)

1. Make *Dessert Crepes*, p. 135.

2. Make *Lemon Pie Filling,* p. 123, steps #2-5, for 9" pie. You will need about 1½ cups of this pudding; cool.

3. For topping, cut up:
   about 3 cups fresh and/or frozen fruit
   (strawberries, bananas, peaches, raspberries)

5. Place 3 tablespoons lemon filling on one side of crepe; roll up and place seam side down on serving plate.

4. If desired briefly warm rolled crepes in 300°-350° oven, uncovered.

5. To serve, top crepes with:
   about 1/3 cup fruit per crepe
   whipped cream

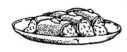

Per 1 filled crepe of 8 with 1/3 cup fruit, whipped cream not included   Exchanges: 0.25 Meat, 0.5 Bread, 1.25 Fat, 0.5 Fruit; 249 Calories, 5 g protein (8%), 8 g fat (28%; g sugars), 41 g carbohydrate (64%; 20 g sugars), 2 g dietary fiber, 82 mg cholesterol, 76 mg sodium, $.45

Banana Cream Crepes

AMOUNT: 8-9 Crepes (4 Servings--2 Each)

1. Make *Vanilla Pudding*, below, using **3 Tbsps. cornstarch**; cool.

2. Make *Dessert Crepes*, p. 135, using the **2 egg whites** leftover from making pudding in place of whole egg.

3. Make *Chocolate Sauce*, p. 156, with **1 - 1 oz. square chocolate.**

4. Fold **1 diced banana** into **1½ cups cooled pudding.**

5. Place 3 tablespoons pudding on one side of crepe; roll up and place on serving plate.

6. If desired briefly warm rolled crepes in 300°-350° oven, uncovered.

7. To serve, top crepes with:
   drizzle of *Chocolate Sauce*
   whipped cream

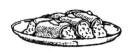

Per 1 filled crepe of 8, sauce and whipped cream not included
  Exchanges: 0.25 Fat, 0.25 Milk, 0.25 Bread, 1 Fat, 0.25 Fruit; 125 Calories,
3.5 g protein (11%), 6 g fat (41%), 16 g carbohydrate (49%; 14 g sugars), 0.5 g dietary fiber,
38 mg cholesterol, 101 mg sodium, $.20

Vanilla Pudding

A simple creamy pudding. Dress it up with a topping or fold in fruit.

AMOUNT: 5 - ½ Cup Servings

1. In saucepan or double boiler (p. 47) whisk together and bring to a low boil for 1 minute over medium heat, whisking constantly:
   2 cups cold nonfat milk *(or alternative, p. 39)*
   2 tablespoons cornstarch or arrowroot powder *(p. 13)*
   3/8 cup crystalline fructose *(p. 13)* **or ¼ cup mild honey** *(p. 24)*
   ¼ teaspoon salt

2. Gradually stir at least half the cooked mixture into egg yolks, whisk back into saucepan with remaining mixture; boil again for 1 minute, remove from heat and stir in butter and vanilla:
   2 slightly beaten egg yolks
   2 tablespoons butter *(unsalted preferred, p. 32)*
   1 teaspoons vanilla

3. Pour into dessert dishes and chill. If desired, top with **toasted sliced almonds** *(p. 73)* **or toasted coconut** *(see under Variation, p. 122)*

Per serving of 5, topping not included
  Exchanges: 0.5 Meat, 0.5 Milk, 0.25 Bread, 1 Fat; 177 Calories, 6 g protein (13%), 7 g fat (35%),
23 g carbohydrate (51%; 20 g sugars), 100 mg cholesterol, 135 mg sodium, $.30

Elegant Fruit Platter

The most colorful and healthful of all desserts! For an extra touch, serve Banana or Persimmon Nut Bread or Scripture Fruit Cake with it.

AMOUNT: See Steps #6, 7

1. Choose an arrangement; here are two suggestions:

circular style

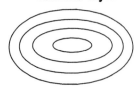

(place dip or cheese cubes in center, optional)

wedge style

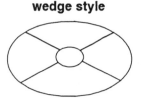

2. Select **3-5 Fruits** with color, shape, and texture contrast:

red	red apple wedges (coat with orange juice *--see #4 below*)
	strawberries (serve whole with tops intact)
	red sweet cherries (leave the stems on)
	red grapes (serve in small clumps with stems)
	watermelon (unpeeled wedges or peeled chunks on toothpicks)
green	Thompson seedless grapes (serve in small clumps with stems)
	kiwi fruit (peeled slices or unpeeled wedges)
	green apple wedges (coat with orange juice--see #4 below)
	honeydew melon (thin wedges, peeled or unpeeled)
yellow	pineapple (cut in thin wedges, or chunks on toothpicks)
	peaches (peel and wedge; with toothpicks, if desired)
	banana (unpeeled chunks--cut banana in 3rds or 4ths; dip cut ends in orange juice--see #4 below)
	papaya (thin wedges, peeled)
cream	bananas (peeled chunks; coat with orange juice--see #4 below) pears (unpeeled wedges; coat with orange juice)
	apples (peeled wedges; coat with orange juice)
orange	oranges (peeled or unpeeled slices, unpeeled wedges)
	cantaloupe (thin wedges peeled or unpeeled)
	nectarines (wedge; serve with toothpicks, if desired)
	persimmons, Fuju or Japanese (unpeeled, sliced) (see p. 108)

3. Have fruits chilled. Wash grapes and unpeeled fruits (see tip, 131).

4. Cut fruits that turn brown from oxidation at last minute (apples, pears, bananas). Dipping in orange juice gives a nice flavor and effectively prevents browning. <u>Cont'd next page</u>

138

5. **Extra Touches:**

Fruit Dip, below; allow 2-3 tablespoons per person
Peanut Butter Dip (blend peanut butter and honey)
Cheese Cubes (contrast with white and yellow cheese; stick cubes on toothpicks into apple in center of serving plate)

6. Calculating Quantities: What you can get out of each piece fruit:
   strawberries - 16-24 berries per 12 oz. box (allow 2-3 per person)
   apples - 6-8 wedges
   cheese cubes - about 120-¾" square cubes per lb.
      (allow 2-3 per person)
   cherries - 3½ cups per lb.
   grapes - 3 cups per lb. or 12-13 clumps per lb.
   watermelon - 30 thin wedges per 12 lb.
   kiwi fruit - 6 slices or wedges
   pineapple - 24-32 wedges per 4 lb. unpeeled fresh
   peaches/nectarines - 6 wedges
   banana - 3 - 4 chunks
   papaya - 10-12 wedges
   pears - 6 wedges
   oranges - 6 slices or 8 wedges
   cantaloupe - 10-20 wedges
   honeydew melon - 20-30 wedges
   Japanese (*Fuju*) persimmons - 6 slices

Sample Fruit Platter for 8

①   1 apple, cut in 8 wedges

②   1 orange, cut in 8 wedges

③   2 bananas, each cut in 4ths

④   10 oz. grapes--8 clumps

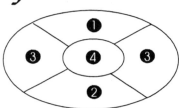

Per serving of Sample Fruit Platter for 8:
  Exchanges: 1.25 Fruit; 77 Calories, 1 g protein (4%), 0.5 g. fat (4%),
19.5 g carbohydrate (92%; 14 g sugars), 2 g dietary fiber, 0 mg cholesterol, 2 mg sodium, $.25

Fruit Dip

Amount: About 2/3 Cup (4-6 Servings)

Whisk together:
    ¼ cup light sour cream or sour cream
    ¼ cup nonfat or lowfat plain yogurt
    3 tablespoons all-fruit spread (any flavor) *(p. 14)*

Per tablespoon with light sour cream, nonfat yogurt
  Exchanges: 0.25 Fruit; 25 Calories, 0.5 g protein (10%), 0.5 g fat (22%),
4 g carbohydrate (68%; 4 g sugars), 2 mg cholesterol, 8 mg sodium, $.10

Banana Nut Bread

A Nut bread served with a tray of fresh fruits or a fresh fruit cocktail makes an elegantly simple dessert or appetizer.

AMOUNT: One Medium Loaf Pan or 3 Mini Loaves *(p. 47)*.
Bake 325° for 60-70 minutes

1. Preheat oven to 325°. Grease or generously spray pan (p. 54).

2. Whisk honey into butter until smooth and creamy; whisk in remaining ingredients:
   ½ stick (¼ cup) soft butter, optional *(unsalted preferred, p. 32)*
   ½ cup honey
   2 eggs *(or alternative, p. 39)*
   1 cup ripe mashed bananas (about 3 small or 2 large bananas)
   ¾ cup buttermilk or pineapple juice, unsweetened (6 oz. can)
   1 teaspoon vanilla

3. Blend dry ingredients in a separate bowl; blend into liquid ingredients just until mixed:
   3 cups whole wheat pastry flour *(p. 14; or alternative, pp. 20-22)*
   3 teaspoons baking powder *(low sodium or Rumford preferred, p. 13)*
   1 teaspoon salt
   ½ teaspoon cinnamon
   ¾ cup chopped walnuts

4. Pour batter into greased loaf pan; bake in preheated oven at 325° for 60-70 minutes or until a knife comes clean out of center.

5. Turn out onto cooking rack or bread board; cool thoroughly. Refrigerate before slicing to minimize crumbling.

Per slice of 16, with 1% fat buttermilk, butter excluded
Exchanges: 0.25 Meat, 1.5 Bread, 0.5 Fat, 0.25 Fruit; 195 Calories,
5.5 g protein (11%), 5 g fat (20%), 37 g carbohydrate (69%; 13 g sugars),
3.5 g dietary fiber, 27 mg cholesterol, 156 mg sodium, $.25

Persimmon Nut Bread

Follow *Banana Nut Bread* recipe above, omitting banana, milk, and vanilla. Add:
   1 - 1½ cups persimmon pulp (2-3 persimmons) *(see tip, p. 126)*
   ½ cup raisins (soak to soften; drain)
   1 teaspoon cinnamon (in place of ½ tsp.)
   ½ teaspoon ground cloves
   ½ teaspoon nutmeg

Per slice of 16, with 1% fat buttermilk, butter excluded   Exchanges: 0.25 Meat, 1.5 Bread, 0.5 Fat, 0.5 Fruit; 209 Calories, 5 g protein (9%), 4.5 g fat (19%), 41 g carbohydrate (72%; 16 g sugars), 4 g dietary fiber, 27 mg cholesterol, 145 mg sodium, $.25

Honey Vanilla Ice Cream

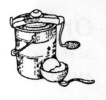

AMOUNT: 2 Quarts

1. Whisk together until well blended:
   4 eggs
   1 cup mild-flavored honey *(p. 25)*
   2 tablespoons vanilla

2. Blend in:
   1 quart lowfat milk
   1 pint (2 cups) whipping cream, unwhipped

3. Process in ice cream maker according to appliance directions or follow *Frozen Vanilla Yogurt*, below, steps # 2-4.

Per ½ cup   Exchanges: 0.25 Meat, 0.25 Milk, 2.25 Fat; 217 Calories 4 g protein (8%),
13.5 g fat (54%), 21 g carbohydrate (38%; 21 g sugars), 99 mg cholesterol, 60 mg sodium, $.35

Frozen Vanilla Yogurt

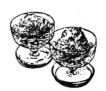

A crunchy ice frost.

AMOUNT: 2 Cups

1. Liquify in blender:
   2 cups nonfat or lowfat plain yogurt
   ¼ cup crystalline fructose *(p. 13)*
   1 teaspoon vanilla

2. Pour into bowl or tray; freeze until set.

3. Scoop into electric mixer; beat until soft.

4. Refreeze until set.

5. Allow to stand at room temperature about 10 minutes before serving.

Per ½ cup with nonfat yogurt   Exchanges: 0.5 Milk; 98 Calories, 6.5 g protein (25%),
19 g carbohydrate (73%; 21 g sugars), 2 mg cholesterol, 67 mg sodium, $.40

Ice Cream Social

Serve **Honey Vanilla Ice Cream** and **Frozen Vanilla Yogurt** with choice of toppings:
   Chocolate or Carob Sauce *(p. 156)*
   Crushed pineapple or Pineappe Topping *(p. 157)*
   Fresh berries or Strawberry Topping *(p. 157)*
   Fresh peach slices
   Carob chips and/or chopped nuts

Orange Ambrosia

So simple to prepare, yet refreshing and tasty!

AMOUNT: 2 Servings

Combine; chill to serve:
> **1 orange, peeled, cut in chunks**
> **1 cup fresh or unsweetened canned pineapple chunks**
> **2 tablespoons raisins**
> **2 tablespoons toasted coconut** *(see under Variation, p. 122)*
> **1 teaspoon crystalline fructose** *(p. 13)*

Per serving of 2   Exchanges: 0.5 Fat, 1.75 Fruit; 142 Calories, 2 g protein (5%), 3 g fat (18%), 30 g carboydrate, (78%; 24 g sugars), 4.5 g dietary fiber, 3 mg. sodium, $.35

Rainbow Chiffon Jello Cubes

Children will love eating and making this! Select juice from the wide variety of frozen unsweetened concentrates now available in supermarkets.

AMOUNT: 8 Servings

1. In saucepan whisk gelatine into water; let stand to soften 5 minutes; bring just to a boil to dissolve:
   > **½ cup cold water** (room temperature okay)
   > **2 envelopes (4 teaspoons) unflavored gelatine** *(p. 15)*

2. Place in blender; puree thoroughly, about 30 seconds:
   > **12 oz. can unsweetened frozen fruit juice concentrate**
   > **1 1/8 cups water**
   > **dissolved gelatine**

3. Pour into a lightly greased 8" or 9" square bake pan.

4. Chill until set. Foamy light colored jello will rise to the top, while darker, clearer jello will remain on the bottom for a two-toned effect.

5. Cut cubes with a sharp knife, 8 x 8.

6. Gently lift out cubes with metal spatula or pancake turner. Fill individual dessert dishes.

Per serving of 8 - 8 jello cubes   Exchanges: 1.5 Fruit; 96 Calories, 2.5 g protein (10%), 22 g carbohydrate (90%; 17 g sugars), 10 mg sodium, $.30

VARIATIONS

~ For clear and dark plain jello cubes without the light colored chiffon effect and texture, do not puree ingredients in the blender.

~ Mix cubes with whipped cream

Strawberry or Peach Shortcake

The traditional with whole grain shortcake. Sometimes we like to serve it a la mode (with frozen yogurt), with or without the whipped cream.

AMOUNT: 9" Square or 9" Pie Pan
Bake 450° for 12-15 minutes, uncovered

1. Stir sweetener into fruit; let stand while preparing shortcake (sugar brings out some of the juices for delectable sweetness):

   6 cups fresh strawberries (about 3--12 oz. boxes) **or peach slices**
   2 tablespoons crystalline fructose *(p. 13)* **or honey**

2. Preheat oven to 450°; generously grease or spray pan (p. 54).

3. Blend together:

   2 cups whole wheat pastry flour *(p. 14; or alternative, pp. 20-22)*
   1 tablespoon crystalline fructose
   3 teaspoons baking powder *(low sodium or Rumford preferred, p. 13)*
   ½ teaspoon salt

4. With pastry blender (p. 49), or 2 table knives cut butter into dry ingredients until crumbly, the size of peas; stir in milk with a fork just until blended (do not overmix):

   1/3 cup soft butter *(unsalted preferred, p. 32)*
   1 cup nonfat milk *(or alternative, p. 39)*

5. Spread dough evenly in pan; Dot with **1 tablespoon butter.**

6. Bake uncovered in preheated oven at 450° for 12-15 minutes.

7. Optional--While cake bakes prepare *Whipped Cream*, p. 155. Refrigerate until ready to serve.

8. To serve: While hot, cut baked shortcake into squares or wedges; split each serving in half. In serving dishes, place prepared fruit between cut halves of cake and over top; top with whipped cream, if desired.

Per serving of 8 with strawberries or peaches, whipped cream not included
   Exchanges: 1.75 Bread, 1.75 Fat, 0.5 Fruit; 264-269 Calories, 5-5.5 g protein (8%),
10 g fat (32%), 43 g carbohydrate (60%; 12 g sugars), 5-5.5 g dietary fiber, 25 mg cholesterol,
138 mg sodium, $.50 Strawberry, $.35 Peach

Fruit Shrub

Colorful, juicy, and refreshing! A 3-minute dessert adapted from the delightful shrub we enjoyed at The Kings Arms Restaurant in Williamsburg, Virginia.

AMOUNT: 10 Servings

1. Chill juices in advance.

2. Blend the juices; divide the sherbert into desert dishes and pour the juice over it in amount desired:
   12 oz. can apricot nectar *(p. 14)*
   12 oz. can unsweetened pineapple juice
   6 oz. can grapefruit juice, unsweetened *(p. 15)*
   2 pints (1 quart) lemon, pineapple, or orange sherbert

3. Serve immediately.

Per serving of 10
   Exchanges: 1 Fruit; 146 Calories, 36 g carbohydrate (98%; 20 g sugars), $.50

Lite Chocolate Pudding

It's "okay" to indulge your love for chocolate--occasionally! This pudding is done in 10 minutes and plenty rich!

AMOUNT: 6 - ½ Cup Servings

1. Whisk together in a medium saucepan or double boiler (p.47):
   ½ cup crystalline fructose *(p. 13)* **or honey**
   6 tablespoons (¼ cup + 2 Tbsp.) cocoa powder *(p. 42 for alternative)*

2. In a 1 quart measuring cup whisk cornstarch into milk until well blended:
   3 cups nonfat milk *(or alternative, p. 39)*
   3½ tablespoons cornstarch *(p. 15)*

3. Gradually whisk milk mixture into dry ingredients in saucepan. Bring to a low boil over medium-high heat, whisking constantly. Continue to whisk and cook at low boil for 2 minutes. Remove from heat.

4. Stir in:
   1 teaspoon vanilla
   dash salt

5. Pour into dessert dishes and chill.

Per serving of 6   Exchanges: 0.5 Milk, 0.5 Bread, 0.25 Fat; 148 Calories, 10 g protein (27%), 1 g fat (6%), 25 g carbohydrate (68%; 23 g sugars), 3 mg cholesterol, 12 mg sodium, $.30

Carob or Chocolate Blanc Mange

A simply delectable pudding and frequent company dessert! Originally made with white sugar and chocolate only, it was a childhood favorite we begged Mother to make often, squabbling over who would get the last bite! Our own children followed suit, although the recipe has changed somewhat for the better nutritionally. A good recipe to introduce carob.

AMOUNT: 8 - ½ Cup Servings

1. Place milk and chocolate (or carob blended smooth with water) in medium saucepan over moderate heat until milk is hot and chocolate melted; do not boil:
   1½ cups lowfat milk
   1 oz. square unsweetened chocolate
   or 2 Tbsps. hot water + 3 Tbsps. carob powder *(p. 13)*
   (stir carob through strainer to remove any lumps)

2. Whisk gelatine into milk in a 1 cup measuring cup; let stand 5 minutes to soften:
   ½ cup cold lowfat milk
   1½ envelopes (3 teaspoons) unflavored gelatine *(p. 15)*

3. Whisk softened gelatine into hot milk mixture; continue to whisk until gelatine is dissoved, about 1 minute. Remove from heat; whisk in:
   ¼ cup mild honey *(p. 25)* **or 1/3 cup crystalline fructose** *(p. 13)*
   1 teaspoon vanilla

4. Pour into mixing bowl; chill until partially set. Do not allow to gel too much or the whipped cream will not blend in easily.

5. Fold in whipped cream. If done carefully without over-mixing, an electric mixer used briefly will do a better job:
   2 cups whipped cream (½ pint heavy cream, whipped)

6. Fill dessert dishes or serving bowl. Return to refrigerator until set.

7. Garnish, if desired, with almonds or coconut.

Per serving of 8 - about ½ cup <u>with chocolate</u>
   Exchanges: 0.25 Milk, 2.5 Fat; 187 Calories, 4 g protein (8%),
14 g fat (64%), 13.5 g carbohydrate (27%; 12 g sugars),
45 mg cholesterol, 42 mg sodium, $.30

Per serving of 8 - about ½ cup <u>with carob</u>
   Exchanges: 0.25 Milk, 2.25 Fat; 180 Calories, 4 gm protein (8%),
12 gm fat (59%), 15 gm carbohydrate (33%; 12 g sugars),
45 mg cholesterol, 43 mg sodium, $.30

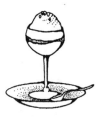

145

Almond Millet Custard

Try this tasty dessert using millet, a most neglected whole grain among Americans!
Serve hot or cold.

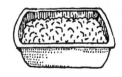

AMOUNT: 6 Servings
Bake 350° for 45-60 minutes, uncovered

1. In a saucepan bring water to a boil, add salt and gradually whisk in millet:
   2 cups water
   ½ teaspoon salt
   ½ cup millet, uncooked grain *(p. 14)*

2. Lower heat to simmering, cover and cook about 40 minutes until cereal is cooked and water completely absorbed.

3. For topping, lightly brown almonds in butter; set aside:
   1 tablespoon melted butter *(unsalted preferred, p. 32)*
   ¼ cup sliced raw almonds *(p. 13)*

4. Grease or spray 8" or 9" square bake pan or 1½ quart casserole dish (p. 54). Preheat oven to 350°.

5. Thoroughly whisk together and pour into baking dish:
   2 eggs, beaten
   1/3 cup honey
   1 cup lowfat milk *(or alternative, p. 39)*
   1 cup water
   2 teaspoons almond extract
   cooked millet (about 2 cups)

6. Top with **lightly toasted almonds** *(see tip, p. 73).*

7. Bake uncovered in preheated oven at 350° for 45-60 minutes until set.

Per serving of 6   Exchanges: 0.5 Meat, 0.25 Milk, 1 Bread, 1 Fat; 215 Calories, 6.5 g protein (11%), 8 g fat (32%), 32.5 g carbohydrate (57%; 17 g sugars), 1.5 g dietary fiber, 79 mg cholesterol, 223 mg sodium, $.35

Vanilla Raisin Custard

Replace almonds and almond extract with:
   1 teaspoon vanilla
   ¼ cup raisins (soften in water; drain)

Per serving of 6   Exchanges: 0.25 Meat, 0.25 Milk, 0.75 Bread, 0.5 Fat, 0.25 Fruit; 200 Calories, 5.5 g protein (10%), 5 g fat (22%), 36 g carbohydrate (68%; 22 g sugars), 1 g dietary fiber, 79 mg cholesterol, 223 mg sodium, $.30

Tapioca Pudding

This has always been one of our family favorites.
Enjoy the texture of the small pearls. Children
especially enjoy tapioca.

AMOUNT: 8 - ½ Cup Servings

1. In medium saucepan or double boiler (p. 47) whisk
   together and bring to a low boil, whisking constantly:
   1/3 cup small pearl tapioca *(p. 14; see About Tapioca below)*
   3 cups nonfat or lowfat milk *(or alternative, p. 39)*
   ¼ teaspoon salt

2. Reduce heat to very low and simmer uncovered for
   5 minutes (stirring constantly is not necessary); while
   simmering, gradually whisk in:
   1/3 cup crystalline fructose *(p. 13)* **or honey**

3. Gradually whisk part of the hot pudding mixture into
   eggs and gradually whisk back into saucepan with
   remaining pudding:
   2 beaten eggs

4. Bring to a boil; boil over lowest possible heat for 5-10 minutes
   while stirring until almost of desired consistency (thickens a bit
   more during cooling).

5. Remove from heat, cool 15 minutes and blend in:
   ½ teaspoon vanilla

6. Pour into dessert dishes; serve warm or chilled.

Per serving of 8, with nonfat milk
   Exchanges: 0.25 Meat, 0.25 Milk, 0.25 Bread; 110 Calories, 5 g protein (18%),
1.5 g fat (14%), 18.5 g carbohydrate (69%; 13 g sugars), 55 mg cholesterol, 85 mg sodium, $.25

Per serving of 8, with lowfat milk
   Exchanges: 0.25 Meat, 0.5 Milk, 0.25 Bread, 0.25 Fat; 121 Calories, 4.5 g protein (15%),
3 g fat (24%), 18.5 g carbohydrate (61%; 13 g sugars), 60 mg cholesterol, 130 mg sodium, $.25

About Tapioca: Tapioca is an easily digested complex starchy carbohydrate from the cassava or manioc plant. Instant or quick-cooking tapioca
is starch baked to remove all the moisture. Pearl tapioca is made by forcing
the starch through various sized sieves. While the whole form may be
considered the most nutritious, it requires soaking for several hours plus
about 1 hour of cooking. Small pearl tapioca, on the other hand, cooks
up in a reasonably short time. It may be purchased at a health food store.

Apricot Yogurt Pudding

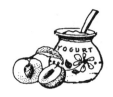

Yogurt and kefir puddings, pp. 148-151, provide a more easily digestible milk protein dessert. Dried fruit especially imparts a fruity flavor.

AMOUNT: 6 Servings

1. Soften fruit in water overnight:
   ¾ cup dried apricots, unsulfured *(p. 13)*
   ¾ cup water

2. Drain the juice from softened apricots into a 1 cup measuring cup; add more water as needed to make **½ cup juice.**

3. In small saucepan whisk gelatine into juice, let stand 5 minutes to soften; dissolve over moderate heat, whisking constantly until just comes to a boil, about 1 minute:
   1 envelope (2 teaspoons) unflavored gelatine *(p. 15)*
   ½ cup juice

4. Place in blender and puree on high speed:
   2 cups nonfat plain yogurt *(or pasteurized alternative, p. 39)*
   2 tablespoons honey or crystalline fructose *(p. 13)*
   softened apricots
   dissolved gelatine

5. Pour into dessert dishes, mold, or serving bowl; chill until set.

Per serving of 6
   Exchanges: 0.25 Bread, 0.75 Fruit; 97 Calories, 6 g protein (22%),
20 g carbohydrate (76%; 29 g sugars), 1 g dietary fiber, 1 mg cholesterol,
46 mg sodium, $.50

Orange Yogurt Pudding

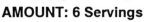

AMOUNT: 6 Servings

1. Use recipe for *Apricot Yogurt Pudding*, above. Omit steps #1, 2..

2. Use **½ cup orange juice** in step #3 in place of apricot juice.

3. Replace apricots with **1 peeled orange** in step #4.

4. Optional--Fold **1 peeled chopped orange** into pureed mixture.

Per serving of 6 using 2 oranges
   Exchanges: 0.25 Milk, 0.5 Fruit; 89 Calories, 6 g protein (25%),
17 g carbohydrate (73%; 18 g sugars), 0.5 g dietary fiber, 1 mg cholesterol, 45 mg sodium, $.30

Spiced Apple Yogurt Pudding

AMOUNT: 6 Servings

1. Follow recipe for *Apricot Yogurt Pudding*,
   p.148, using apples in place of apricots;
   soak overnight:
   ½ cup dried apples, unsulfured *(p.13)*
   ¾ cup water
2. Add in step #4:
   ½ teaspoon cinnamon
   1/8 teaspoon nutmeg

Per serving of 6
   Exchanges: 0.25 Milk, 0.25 Fruit; 79 Calories, 5.5 g protein (25%),
15 g carbohydrate (72%; 17 g sugars), 0.5 g dietary fiber, 1 mg cholesterol, 45 mg sodium, $.35

Pineapple Yogurt Pudding

AMOUNT: 6 Servings

1. Follow recipe for *Apricot Yogurt Pudding*,
   p. 148. Omit steps #1,2.

2. Drain **8 oz. can crushed pineapple, reserving the juice**.

3. Use **reserved pineapple juice** in step #3 in place of apricot juice.

4. Do not use blender. Whisk ingredients together until
   smooth replacing apricots with **drained pineapple**.

Per serving of 6
   Exchanges: 0.25 Milk, 0.25 Fruit; 82 Calories, 5.5 g protein (25%),
16 g carbohydrate (73%; 17 g sugars), 1 mg cholesterol, 48 mg sodium, $.30

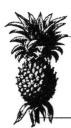

> **About Pineapple with Gelatine** Do not use fresh pineapple
> with gelatine. The enzymic action of fresh pineapple will
> inactivate its gelling action. Always used canned pineapple
> for gelatine desserts or salads.

Strawberry Kefir Pudding

Another tasty dessert made with a cultured milk that is easier on the digestion, yet high in protein. Kefir may be purchased at some health food stores. See **Breakfasts**, *p. 32.*

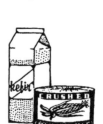

AMOUNT: 4 Servings

1. In small saucepan whisk gelatine into water, let stand 5 minutes to soften; dissolve over moderate heat, whisking constantly, about 1 minute:
   ¼ cup cold water (or room temperature)
   1 envelope (2 teaspoons) unflavored gelatine *(p. 15)*

2. Place in blender and puree:
   1 cup *Strawberry Kefir* *(p. 13)*
   1 cup strawberries, fresh or frozen, unsweetened
   1 tablespoon honey or crystalline fructose *(p. 13)*
   dissolved gelatine

3. Pour into individual dessert dishes or serving bowl; chill until set.

4. Garnish servings, if desired, with **fresh strawberry** and **mint leaf.**

Per serving of 4; garnish not included
Exchanges: 0.25 Milk, 0.25 Fat, 0.25 Fruit; 82 Calories, 4 g protein (18%), 2.5 g fat (24%), 13 g carbohydrate (58%; 14 g sugars), 0.5 g dietary fiber, 7 mg cholesterol, 27 mg sodium, $.30

Pineapple Kefir Pudding

AMOUNT: 4 Servings

1. Follow recipe for ***Strawberry Kefir Pudding***, above, replacing strawberry kefir and strawberries with:
   1 cup *Pineapple Kefir* *(p. 13)*
   8 oz. can crushed pineapple, unsweetened

2. Drain pineapple; use the drained juice in place of water to soften and dissolve gelatine.

3. Whisk or stir drained pineapple and sweetener together instead of blending in blender.

Per serving of 4
Exchanges: 0.25 Milk, 0.25 Fat, 0.75 Fruit; 106 Calories, 4 g protein (14%), 2 g fat (18%), 19 g carbohydrate (68%; 15 g sugars), 0.5 g dietary fiber, 7 mg cholesterol, 32 mg sodium, $.30

Peach Kefir Pudding

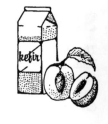

AMOUNT: 4 Servings

Follow recipe for **Strawberry Kefir Pudding**,
p. 150, using in place of strawberry kefir
and strawberries:

> **1 cup *Peach Kefir*** *(p. 13)*
> **1 cup chopped fresh peaches, peeled**

Per serving of 4 using 2 medium peaches
> *Exchanges: 0.25 Milk, 0.25 Fat, 0.5 Fruit 90 Calories, 4 g protein (16%), 2.5 g fat (23%),*
> *15 g carbohydrate (61%; 11 g sugars), 0.5 g dietary fiber, 7 mg cholesterol, 27 mg sodium, $.30*

Old Fashioned Rice Pudding

A tasty way to use leftover brown rice. Enjoy cold or hot.

AMOUNT: 6 Servings
Bake 350° for about 1 hour, uncovered

1. Preheat oven to 350°.

2. In 1½ quart casserole dish whisk honey into eggs;
   whisk in remaining ingredients, adding milk last:

   > **2 eggs, beaten well**
   > **¼ cup honey**
   > **1 cup cooked brown rice** *(p. 14; see Note below)*
   > **½ cup raisins**
   > **1 teaspoon vanilla**
   > **1 teaspoon lemon extract**
   > **½ teaspoon nutmeg**
   > **¼ teaspoon salt**
   > **2 cups lowfat milk** *(or alternative, p. 39)*

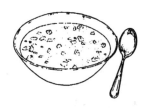

Per serving of 6
> *Exchanges: 0.25 Meat, 0.5 Milk, 0.25 Fat, 0.5 Fruit*
> *184 Calories, 6 g protein (13%), 3.5 g fat (18%),*
> *33 g carbohydrate (70%; 24 g sugars), 1 g dietary fiber,*
> *77 mg cholesterol, 244 mg sodium, $.35*

Note To cook brown rice, see **Main Dishes**, p. 206, or **Casseroles**, p. 65.

Sweet 'n Spicy Pudding

This incredibly rich, and delicious, dessert turns your failures into success. I often make this with failed homemade bread, or with leftover or over-baked bran muffins. Make servings small. Serve with Whipped Cream or Lemon Sauce.

AMOUNT: 8 Servings
Bake 300° for 60-75 minutes, uncovered

1. Preheat oven to 300°. Grease or spray a 1½ quart casserole dish or oven-proof bowl with non-stick spray (p. 54).

2. Whisk all ingredients together in order given in the greased or sprayed casserole dish:
   - **1 stick (½ cup) melted butter** *(unsalted preferred, p. 32)*
   - **¾ cup honey** (in a double recipe use 1 cup only), whisk thoroughly into melted butter until smooth and creamy
   - **1 egg** *(or alternative, p. 39)*
   - **1 cup nonfat milk** *(or alternative, p. 39)*
   - **2 cups dry whole grain bread crumbs** *(see Dry Bread Tip below)*
     or 3-3½ cups soft bread, crumbled
     or 6 bran muffins, crumbled
   - **½ cup raisins, chopped dates** *(see tip, p. 71)* **or date nuggets** *(p. 13)*
   - **½ cup coarsely chopped walnuts**
   - **1 teaspoon cinnamon**
   - **½ teaspoon ground cloves**
   - **½ teaspoon nutmeg**
   - **1 teaspoon baking soda**
   - **½ teaspoon salt**

3. Bake uncovered in preheated oven at 300° for 30 minutes. Stir pudding thoroughly to reblend ingredients. Bake 30-45 minutes longer until dark brown.

4. Serve warm or cold in dessert dishes topped, if desired, with **Whipped Cream** or **Lemon Sauce**, p. 155.

Per serving of 8, using 4 slices soft bread; topping not included   Exchanges: 0.25 Meat, 0.75 Bread, 3 Fat, 0.5 Fruit; 335 Calories, 6 g protein (7%), 17 g fat (44%), 44 g carbohydrate (50%; 35 g sugars), 3 g dietary fiber, 58 mg cholesterol, 338 mg sodium, $.40

> **Dry Bread Tip:** Lay bread slices in single layer, uncovered, in open air until dried out (this can take several days); crumble. Store crumbs in a tightly closed freezer bag in freezer until ready to use.

Sauces & Toppings

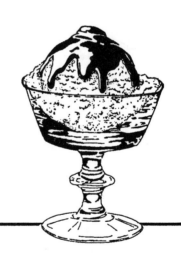

*Everyone brings out the choice wine first
and then the cheaper wine after the guests
have had too much to drink;
but you have saved the best till now.*
John 2:10

Sauces & Toppings

Lemon Sauce

A little goes a long way. Serve over unfrosted cakes. Sauce thickens as it cools.

AMOUNT: 1 Cup (6 - 8 Servings)

1. Blend together in a saucepan:
   1 cup water
   1½ tablespoons cornstarch or arrowroot powder *(p. 13)*
   ¼ cup crystalline fructose *(p. 13)* **or mild-flavored honey** *(p. 25)*
   ¼ cup lemon juice (preferrably fresh)
   1 egg
   2 tablespoons butter *(unsalted preferred, p. 32)*
   2 teaspoons grated lemon peel *(see tip, p. 106)*

2. Bring to a boil, stirring constantly with whisk until thickened, about 1 minute.

3. Store in refrigerator; to serve, rewarm over low heat, if desired.

Per tablespoon   Exchanges: 0.25 Fat; 33 Calories, 2 g fat (47%),
4 g carbohydrate (48%; 35 g sugars), 17 mg cholesterol, 5 mg sodium, $.05

Whipped Cream

After reading the ingredients labels of Cool Whip and on pressurized cans of whipped cream or substitutes, I hope you agree with me that the real stuff is a better choice!

AMOUNT: 2 Cups

Whip cream on high speed with electric mixer for about 30 seconds (caution: if overwhipped it will turn to butter); add sweetener and continue to whip until thickened:
   ½ pint (1 cup) heavy whipping cream
      (pp. 14, 15; raw certified preferred, p. 39))
   2 tablespoons crystalline fructose *(p. 13)*
   or mild-flavored honey *(p. 25)*

Per 2 tablespoons   Exchanges: 1 Fat; 57 Calories, 5.5 g fat (84%),
2 g carbohydrate (14%; 2 g sugars), 20 mg cholesterol, 6 mg sodium, $.05 - $.10

> **Freezing Whipped Cream Tip:** Leftover whipped cream can be frozen in dollops on cookie sheet; when frozen, wrap in plastic wrap and store in a tightly covered container. These will keep fresh up to 2 months. For more tips on buying, storing, and preparing whipped cream, see **Keeping Foods Fresh** by Janet Baily, pp. 138-139, an excellent resource book for all natural foods storage.

Chocolate Sauce

AMOUNT: About 1 Cup

1. In saucepan over very low heat melt:
   ½ stick (¼ cup) butter *(unsalted preferred, p. 32)*
   1 or 2 - 1 oz. squares unsweetened chocolate, to taste

2. Whisk in, bring to a boil, whisking constantly until thickened, about 3 minutes:
   1/3 cup crystalline fructose *(p. 13)* **or honey**
   ½ cup evaporated skim milk *(or alternative, p. 39)*

3. Remove from heat; whisk in:
   ½ teaspoon vanilla

Per tablespoon with 1 oz. chocolate   Exchanges: 1 Fat; 64 Calories; 1 g protein (5%),
4.5 g fat (57%), 6 g carbohydrate (37%; 5 g sugars), 9 mg cholesterol, 11 mg sodium, $.10

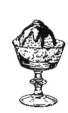

Carob Sauce

AMOUNT: About 1 Cup

1. Follow recipe for **Chocolate Sauce**, above, using in place of chocolate:
   6 tablespoons carob powder *(p. 13)*
   (stir through strainer to remove any lumps)
   ¼ cup hot water

2. Blend carob into hot water; remove melted butter from heat; add carob mixture and remaining ingredients; return to heat to thicken.

Per tablespoon   Exchanges: 0.25 Bread, 0.5 Fat; 58 Calories, 1 g protein (5%),
3 g fat (43%), 8 g carbohydrate (52%; 5 g sugars), 8 mg cholesterol, 10 mg sodium, $.10

Chocolate Carob Sauce

AMOUNT: About 1 Cup

1. Follow recipe for **Chocolate Sauce**, above, using:
   1 - 1 oz. square unsweetened chocolate
   ¼ cup carob powder *(p. 13)*
   2 tablespoons hot water

2. Blend carob with water before adding to the butter.

Per tablespoon   Exchanges: 0.75 Fat; 63 Calories, 1 g protein (5%), 4 g fat (51%),
7 g carbohydrate (44%; 5 g sugars), 8 mg cholesterol, 10 mg sodium, $.10

Pineapple Topping

Serve over unfrosted Carrot Cake, Applesauce Cake, or Date-Nut Cake in place of frosting, or over Honey Vanilla Ice Cream or Frozen Yogurt.

AMOUNT: 1 Cup

1. In saucepan whisk together and cook over low heat, whisking constantly, until thickened (take care--pineapple burns easily):

  8 oz. can crushed pineapple, unsweetened, undrained
  2 teaspoons cornstarch or arrowroot powder *(p. 13)*
  1½ teaspoons honey or crystalline fructose *(p. 13)*

2. Serve hot or cold.

Per tablespoon
  Exchanges: 0.25 Fruit; 12 Calories, 3 g carbohydrate (98%; 2.5 g sugars), 1 mg sodium, $.05

Strawberry Topping

Serve over unfrosted Angel Food Cake, Honey Cheesecake, Lemon Tofu Pie, Yogurt Pie, Honey Vanilla Ice Cream or Frozen Yogurt. I usually use a 12 oz. tub of fresh strawberries for this, but unsweetened frozen strawberries can also be used.

AMOUNT: About 1½ Cups

1. In saucepan whisk together and cook over low heat, whisking constantly, until thickened and clear:

  about ½ cup strawberries, fresh or frozen, crushed
  about ½ cup cold water
  2 tablespoons cornstarch or arrowroot powder *(p. 13)*
  1-2 tablespoons honey or crystalline fructose, to taste *(p. 13)*

2. Stir in:

  1½ cups fresh or frozen strawberries, quartered

3. Serve hot or cold.

Per ¼ Cup using 1 Tbsp. honey
  Exchanges: 0.25 Bread, 0.25 Fruit; 35 Calories, 8.5 g carbohydrate (92%; 5 g sugars), 1 g dietary fiber, 1 mg sodium, $.20

VARIATIONS

In place of strawberries use any other berries desired such as **blueberries, blackberries, raspberries, boysenberries.**

Joy's 4-in-1 Non-Dairy Sauce

A tasty sauce to serve over cakes and scones. This versatile non-dairy recipe with slight variations (p. 159) can also be turned into 2 puddings or a very low sugar, non-dairy frosting for cakes or sweet rolls!

AMOUNT: About 3 Cups

1. **Gelled Fruit Juice**--Soften gelatine in water; bring to boil to dissolve; whisk in honey; remove from heat; stir in juice; chill until firm:
    - **1 cup water** (room temperature)
    - **1 envelope (2 teaspoons) unflavored gelatine** *(p. 15)*
    - **1 teaspoon honey**
    - **1 cup red berry juice or other desired flavor**
      (¼ cup frozen concentrate + ¾ cup water, if desired)

2. **Tofu Beverage Sauce**--Blend and whisk oil, flour, and cornstarch over low heat until smooth and bubbly; remove from heat; whisk in honey and tofu beverage a little at a time until smooth; add salt; return to moderate heat and whisk constantly until thickened, about 1 minute; remove from heat; stir in vanilla; cool:
    - **2 tablespoons canola oil** *(preferred, p. 32)*
    - **2 tablespoons whole wheat pastry** *(p. 14; or alternative, pp. 20-22)*
      or unbleached white flour
    - **2 tablespoons cornstarch**
    - **2 tablespoons mild-flavored honey** *(p. 13)*
    - **1 cup *Better Than Milk Tofu Beverage* *(p. 39)*, reconstituted**
      (2 level Tbsps. powder mixed with water to make 1 cup)
    - **¼ teaspoon salt**
    - **¾ teaspoon vanilla**

3. Whip **Gelled Fruit Juice** (#1 above) in electric mixer until foamy. Remove to another bowl.

4. Whip cooled **Tofu Beverage Sauce** (#2 above) in electric mixer until smooth.

5. Add whipped **Gelled Fruit Juice** to whipped **Tofu Beverage Sauce** in electric mixer. Mix briefly until well blended. Fold in and serve immediately:
    - **1 cup fresh or frozen berries** (or amount desired)

About ¼ Cup 4-in-1 Non-Dairy Sauce or ¼ Cup Berry Non-Dairy Pudding (½ serving, p. 159)
    Exchanges: 0.25 Bread, 0.5 Fat, 0.25 Fruit; 68 Calories, 1 g prtoen (5%), 3 g fat (36%), 10.5 g carbohydrate (59%; 6 g sugars), 0.5 g dietary fiber, 0 mg cholesterol, 56 mg sodium, $.20

¼ Cup (½ serving) Maple Non-Dairy Pudding or Maple Frosting (higher figures) , p. 159
    Exchanges: 0.5 Bread, 1.5 Fat; 137 (145) Calories, 1 g protein (2-3%), 8.5 g fat (50-52%), 16.5 (18) g carbohydrate (46-48%; 9 g sugars - pudding; 18 g sugars--frosting), 0.5 g dietary fiber, 0 mg cholesterol, 164 mg sodium, $.20

Berry Non-Dairy Pudding

Chill **Tofu Beverage Sauce** (step #2) in refrigerator before whipping it and mixing it with **Gelled Fruit Juice** (steps #4, 5). Fill pudding dishes with sauce and chill again thoroughly until further set. If desired, substitute another fruit juice and fruit for berry juice and berries, such as orange-pineapple-banana juice with sliced bananas. 6 - ½ cup servings.

Maple Non-Dairy Pudding

Double the recipe for **Tofu Beverage Sauce** only (step #2), but use **3 Tbsps. each flour and cornstarch**; replace vanilla with **1 tsp. maple flavoring**; fill pudding dishes; chill thoroughly. 4 - ½ cup servings.

Maple Frosting

Make **Tofu Beverage Sauce** only (step #2); replace vanilla with **½-¾ tsp. maple flavoring, to taste**. For cake frosting, chill thoroughly, then whisk or whip until smooth (step #4). For sweet roll frosting, sauce may be whisked or whipped and spread on hot rolls immediately without chilling. Frosts 1 dozen cupcakes or 8-9" square cake, or 1-2 dozen sweet rolls.

Whipped Topping

The spartan low calorie, nonfat alternative to Whipped Cream! Lemon juice helps to stablize it and to minimize the powdered milk taste. This topping should be made and refrigerated no longer than one hour before serving as it will gradually lose fluff, even refrigerated.

AMOUNT: About 3½ Cups

Place water in mixing bowl and chill with electric beaters in freezer until ice begins to form, about 20-30 minutes; add milk powder and beat at high speed until peaks form, about 5 minutes; whip in remaining ingredients, adding sweetener gradually; chill:

>   **½ cup water**
>   **1/3 cup non-instant nonfat dry milk powder** *(p. 14)*
>   **or ½ cup instant dry milk powder**
>   **3 tablespoons lemon juice** *(fresh preferred)*
>   **2 tablespoons crystalline fructose** *(p. 13)* **or honey, to taste**
>   **1 teaspoon vanilla**

Per ¼ cup   Exchanges: negligable; 18 Calories, 1 g protein (23%),
3.5 g carbohydrate (75%; 4 g sugars), 1 mg cholesterol, 16 mg sodium, $.05

The Best Comes Last

. . .you have saved the best till now.   John 2:10

Desserts is the sixth book in our basic series of cookbooks--featuring those delicious treats served at the end of the meal. The best of our lives will come at the end, too, or the worst, depending on how we prepare for it.

The Bible indicates that human history is coming to a close. Jesus Christ is returning to earth soon to establish his eternal kingdom--the new heaven and new earth. In this kingdom peace and righteousness will reign. *The lion will lie down with the lamb* and *swords will be beaten into plowshares.* There will be no more wars. There will be no more sickness. There will be no more heartaches. There will be no more broken relationships. There will be no more bad habits. There will be no more tears. There will be no more death. Every good thing we sought in this life but could not quite experience or attain will be there. . . all those *spiritual riches in the heavenly places.* It will be beyond the richest dessert imaginable in this life. . .*as it is written, 'No eye has seen, nor ear has heard, no mind has conceived what God has prepared for those who love him.' (1 Corinthians 2:9; Isaiah 64:4).*

There will be no need for the eternal God, our Heavenly Father, to rule his kingdom as an earthly dictator does. Having put their complete trust in God to rule in their lives, all the nations of his kingdom will have hearts transformed to live out and do his will voluntarily. How has this been made possible? Only through Jesus Christ. *Salvation is found in no one else, for there is no other name under heaven given to men by which we must be saved (Acts 4:12).* No one in all of human history paid the acceptable price for our ungodliness except God himself in the Person of his son, Jesus. Through faith in him a person receives the Holy Spirit empowering him to live according to the will of God. No religious leader or religious or political system can transform the human heart except Jesus Christ.

God has clearly revealed his transcendent existence, his character, and his power through what he has created. The recognition of the complex nutritional values and taste delights of food alone speaks this message loud and clear. . . *what may be known about God is plain. . . because God has made it plain. . . .For since the creation of the world God's invisible qualities--his eternal power and divine nature--have been clearly seen, being understood from what has been made, so that men are without excuse (Romans 1:19-20).*

Since God has given us such powerful evidence of himself in the creation there remains only the fearful prospect of his judgement if we neglect the great salvation he has provided for us through the sacrifice of His Son. *The God who made the world and everything in it is the Lord of heaven and earth. . . he himself gives all men life and breath and everything else. From one man he made every nation of men, that they should inhabit the whole earth, and he determined the times set for them and the exact places where they should live. God did this so that men would seek him and perhaps reach out for him and find him, though he is not far from each one of us. . .he has set a day when he will judge the world with justice by the man he has appointed. He has given proof of this to all men by raising him from the dead (Acts 17:24-31).* Jesus' resurrection is a well documented historical fact.

But God does not take persons for his kingdom by force. He seeks to win them by love. *Greater love has no one than this, that one lay down his life for his friends (John 15:13).* Jesus Christ laid down his life for us according to the eternal plan and will of God. *God made him who had no sin to be sin for us, so that in him we might become the righeousness of God (2 Corinthians 5:21).* Yet God will not make us believe. God will not make us follow his Son, Jesus, nor make us put our trust in him. But He has done everything, and more, to invite us to do so, to make it possible, and to make it the best for us.

> *And this is the will of him who sent me,*
> *that I shall lose none of all that he has given me,*
> *but raise them up at the last day.*
> *For my Father's will is that everyone*
> *who looks to the Son and believes in him*
> *shall have eternal life,*
> *and I will raise him up at the last day.*
> *John 6:39-40*

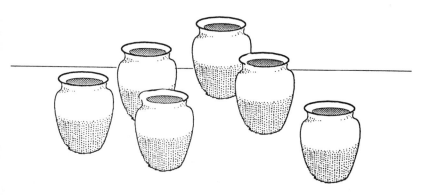

Index

CUT-OUT TABS

CONTENTS	PLANNING	CAKES	PIES

COOKIES & CANDIES	COOKIES	{ alternative shorter title

PUDDINGS & DESSERTS	DESSERTS	{ alternative shorter title

SAUCES & TOPPINGS	INDEX

SAUCES	TOPPINGS	{ alternative shorter titles

Cut on dotted lines. Fold each tab in half.

Overlap tabs about ¼" on each side of divider pages:

Tape tab to page on both sides; tape over entire tab to reinforce. Use magic stick scotch tape for best results.

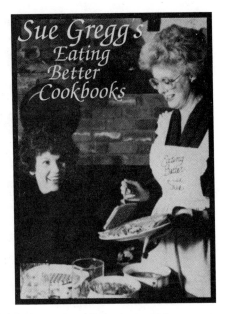

A fter a family health crisis Sue Gregg began to question how to put nutritional value back into family meals.

Nine months of endurance on a rigorous healthfood diet and too many yucks from her family convinced her that few meat and potatoes, biscuits and gravy Americans would survive drastic dietary changes.

Sue began to ask, how could good taste and optimal nutrition go together? Was it possible to transform the quality of ingredients in old favorite family recipes?

She began experimenting with whole food alternatives to white flour, sugar, and hydrogenated fats. Her husband and children complimented successful recipes with yums. Others soon requested recipes and cooking classes.

Sue Gregg is keenly aware of people's food preferences. At age 17 she supervised cooking at a church retreat. During her college years she managed food service for student conferences and international student house parties. For seven summers she fed hundreds of finicky junior highers, high schoolers, collegians, and families at Campus By The Sea on Catalina Island. There was no electricity, freezer, telephone, or road. Supplies arrived via barge.

In a quest for recipes that balance convenience and cost, nutrition and appetite appeal Sue's experimental cooking continues. The testimony to good taste extends from her famous lentil-rice "dog food" casserole to allergy alternative multi-grained blender batter waffles, pancakes, muffins, coffee cakes, and crepes.

Her goal is to help people overcome obstacles to eating better and to benefit from a personal relationship with the Provider of food. She develops resources that enable others to serve a needy world more effectively in better health and with more energy.

In the fall of 1994 she was invited to teach food preparation and nutritional survival skills to American CoMission team members in St. Petersburg and Moscow. Russian teachers also invited her to give demonstrations in their classrooms.

Sue Gregg is the author of more than 13 cookbooks published by Eating Better Cookbooks and Harvest House. She also conducts *Taste & Tell* demonstration workshops with her husband.

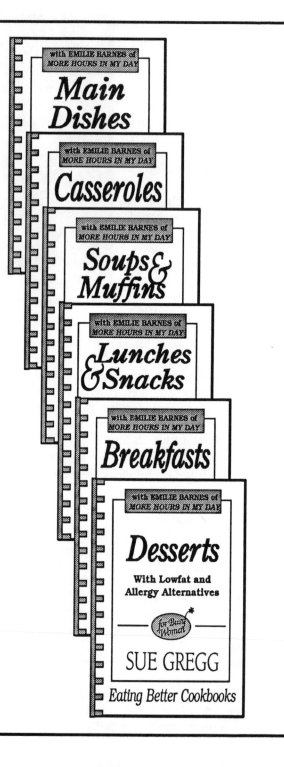

with EMILIE BARNES of
MORE HOURS IN MY DAY

*Main
Dishes*

with EMILIE BARNES of
MORE HOURS IN MY DAY

Casseroles

with EMILIE BARNES of
MORE HOURS IN MY DAY

*Soups&
Muffins*

with EMILIE BARNES of
MORE HOURS IN MY DAY

*Lunches
&Snacks*

with EMILIE BARNES of
MORE HOURS IN MY DAY

Breakfasts

with EMILIE BARNES of
MORE HOURS IN MY DAY

Desserts

**With Lowfat and
Allergy Alternatives**

*for Busy
Women*

SUE GREGG

Eating Better Cookbooks

The Eating Better Cookbooks--Basic Set

Main Dishes includes over 270 recipes and 138 menus. 52 low budget meals. 61 low fat meals average just 20% fat (of calories). Menus include all food groups with vegetarian options. Nutritional data for exchanges, calories, carbohydrate, protein, fat, and fiber. Satisfies the meat and potatoes appetite. Index, 292 pages.

Casseroles stocks your freezer with 5 sets of 5 recipes. A lifesaver when time and energy are short. Now you can say dinner's ready in minutes. Double, triple, quadruple recipes. Includes menus, shopping, and assembly lists. Chicken, fish, ground turkey, bean & vegetarian recipes. A wholefoods convenience cookbook for singles as well as families. Index. 90 pages.

Soups & Muffins provides an easy way to get whole grain variety. 24 muffin recipes from 12 whole grains. Alternatives for wheat & dairy. 27 favorite soup recipes nutritionally improved. Soup and muffin combination menus save $$. Index. 102 pages.

Lunches & Snacks includes a special 75 page guide for young cooks in preparing beverages, breads, crackers, chips, dips, sandwiches, soups, and spreads from set up to clean up. Recipes written by-the-numbers avoid confusion. Nutrition quizzes for discussion. Children learn to master basic kitchen skills with the nutritional why's and prepare complete meals by their teens. Index. 168 pages.

Breakfasts gives you incredibly easy fresh whole grain three minute blender batters for light and tender waffles and pancakes, coffee cakes, muffins, and crepes. Now you can enjoy whole grain nutrition without a grain mill. Introduces Kamut, the versatile allergy alternative grain of the 90's. Includes cinnamon rolls, banana smoothie, cereals, egg variations, fruit dishes, toppings and spreads. wheat, dairy, and egg allergy alternatives. Whole grains researched. Tips for teaching children. Index. 312 pages.

Desserts satisfies the sweet tooth without white flour, white sugar, or hydrogenated fats. Enjoy familiar favorites along with Poppy seed Cake and Sweet n' Spicy Pudding plus alternatives for both chocolate and carob. Whole grain Angel Food Cake at 0% fat. Allergy alternative ingredients included. 45 recipes under 200 calories and 30% fat. Index. 175 pages.

Master Index & Menu Planner (not illustrated) references all six volumes and currently published works so you can find recipes and research subjects quickly. Recipes categorized by type for monthly menu planning. Plan a month's menus in 20 minutes to save time, cost, and what-to-have-for-dinner frustration. Ideal for introducing young cooks to planning menu variety.

The Eating Better Cooking Course

The 15 Minute Meal PLANNER

Eating Better with Sue

The Author of *The Eating Better Cookbooks* shows you how to select and prepare quality whole food ingredients to maximize nutritional benefits and good taste.

Models wholesome food preparation. Explains the reasons for choosing quality alternative ingredients for white sugar, white flour, and hydrogenated shortening. Comprehensible for children but challenging enough for adults. Avoids overwhelming academic technicalities. Motivates to action.

The 15-Minute Meal Manager, A Realistic Approach to a Healthy Lifestyle (Harvest House) addresses concerns about nutrition and taste, cost and convenience. Explains how to get started and how to deal with family resistance to change. Contrasts Biblical and New Age Perspectives on food. More than 50 quick-reading chapters provide a wealth of practical ideas on food selection, preparation and storage along with a starter set of basic recipes using whole ingredients. 384 pages.

The *Eating Better with Sue* video demonstrates Sue Gregg's secrets for light 'n tender whole grain muffins, maximizing flavor and nutrients in soups, convenient casseroles, seasoning ground turkey, sunshine shake, brown rice and more. In step-by-step manner it not only demonstrates recipes but also provides the reasons for choosing ingredients of high nutritional quality. Recipes served with menus in dining settings to conclude each scene. Provides models and motivators for young cooks. Lends authority to mother's teaching about healthier eating. Six segments. 74 minutes.

The Eating Better Cooking Course Workbook and Leader's Guide (not pictured) coordinate video and text lessons with kitchen activities. Recipe evaluation guides. Bible readings. Graduation banquet finale. Appropriate for teaching adults and children.